Nutritional Testing
For
Kinesiologists
And
Dowsers

ISBN: 978-0-9542439-5-1

Published by:

Life-Work Potential Limited
Sea View House
Long Rock
Penzance
Cornwall
TR20 8JF
England

Tel: + 44 (0)1736 719030
Fax: + 44 (0)1736 719040
www.lifeworkpotential.com

Nutritional Testing
For
Kinesiologists
And
Dowsers

Jane Thurnell-Read

Other books by the author:

Verbal Questioning Skills For Kinesiologists
ISBN: 978-0-9542439-1-3, Life-Work Potential, 2004

Energy Mismatch
ISBN: 978-0-9542439-3-7, Life-Work Potential, 2004

Allergy A To Z
ISBN: 978-0-9542439-2-0, Life-Work Potential, 2005

Geopathic Stress
ISBN: 978-0-9542439-4-4 Life-Work Potential, 2006

Health Kinesiology: The Muscle Testing System That Talks To The Body
ISBN 978-0-9542439-6-8, Life-Work Potential Limited, 2009

Visit

www.healthandgoodness.com
for
information, tips and inspiration
for a happier, healthier life

and

Visit

www.lifeworkpotential.com
for
kinesiology test kits
and books by Jane Thurnell-Read

Introduction

This book started out in life as a workshop for kinesiologists. I was struck that a lot of practitioners had completed some nutrition training, but could not see how to integrate it into their sessions with clients. In consequence many were offering very little nutritional advice. So I set out to design a workshop that would teach them this very special skill. The workshop was very successful, but eventually I decided to stop teaching and concentrate on writing and other projects. A book based on the material from that course was a natural outcome of that decision.

This book is different from most nutrition books. It does not set out to teach you a lot of nutrition knowledge and facts. It sets out to teach you how to use your skills as a dowser or kinesiologist in the most effective way possible in this important area. Inevitably, in doing this, I will be presenting some nutritional knowledge, but this is not the main aim of the book. This is a companion book to all the information-dense books you have on nutrition already. This book alone is not enough for you to give sound advice to your clients on nutrition, supplements and diets, but it will allow you to access and act on this information in an efficient and comprehensive manner.

One of the fundamentals of kinesiology and dowsing is that everyone is individual. Of course, we do share much in common – our genetic makeup ensures that – but the variations in what is right for people are significant. This is particularly true in the area of nutrition and diet. Because of this, nutritional knowledge can only be a guide not a prescription. Putting nutritional knowledge together with kinesiology or dowsing provides an amazingly accurate and versatile system.

As ever, the real test of our work is what happens to real people in the real world. I hope that this book will give you the confidence to go out there and do it.

Using this book practically means that you will be using verbal questioning. My book *Verbal Questioning Skills For Kinesiologists* gives a lot more information on how to perfect your verbal questioning skills.

How To Use This Book

I have written this book to be used practically in a particular way. Faced with a client I envisage you will go through the following stages:

1. You decide on which way you will work (see pages 11 to 14).

2. You test from the nutritional menu (pages 25 to 34).

3. Having found a category (in bold with a number against it), read the different possibilities listed below the bold entry. If you have been using this system for a while, or know a lot about nutrition and nutritional testing you may feel able to test straight away. Otherwise, go to (4)

4. Turn to the correct pages and read what it has to stay before testing. You may also want to refer to other books and manuals too. Remember the nutritional information in this book is not intended to be comprehensive or sufficient in its own right.

Walking Your Talk

As with so many other aspects of our life, it is important to walk our talk in respect of our own diet and nutrition.

For many years I was an avid tea drinker – I drank far more than was good for me, but I did not want to stop. Because I was not prepared to reduce or eliminate my tea consumption, I was not prepared to recommend this to clients either. I subconsciously excluded this from my testing, although I would say vaguely to clients sometimes something like: "It seems like a lot of tea isn't likely to be good for your health, so you might like to think about cutting down." Obviously a really positive and clear message! Eventually I realised that I needed to cut down on tea not only for my own sake, but also for the sake of all my clients. Once I had done that I was able to add the possibility of drinking less/no tea into the equation for my clients.

Doing what you advise is also important for other reasons. It is clear to me from teaching students to muscle test for nutritional advice that if your own diet is poor your energy knowledge of a good diet is likely to be poor too. As you improve your own diet, you will be better at testing for the subtle nuances that are needed by different individuals. You will also have more practical knowledge about a whole range of nutritional issues. Encouraging a client to try a particular fruit because you know it tastes good, can massively increase compliance.

The best reason of all for sorting out your diet and nutrition is, of course, that you will almost certainly as a result live a healthier, happier life. We often think of the quality of our diet affecting our health, but it also has a profound effect on our happiness. It has an indirect effect in that if you have arthritis or migraine as a result of what you eat, it will be difficult to be happy. It also has a direct effect too. For example, the B vitamins, and the minerals calcium and magnesium directly affect our moods, and shortages can lead to anxiety, insomnia and palpitations. A student once said to me that she was only attending my nutrition course because she had to in order to meet the requirements of the professional association. She told me she was not interested in nutrition – she was interested in psychological issues. I tried to explain to her that diet and nutrition impacts on all areas of our lives, and that she was doing her clients a disservice if she was not prepared to recognise this. I tried to convince her, I think without success, that she needed to know something about nutrition in order at the very least to be able to refer clients on to a practitioner who was interested in this topic. I also thought she would benefit from knowing more about nutrition for herself, so that she could have the information she needed to make the right choices for herself.

Nutritional Knowledge

Nutritional knowledge is important, and if you want to do good work in this area, you need to spend time understanding the existing information provided by science, medicine, naturopathy, etc.

It is important to study nutrition – I see this as a way of calibrating our measuring instruments – muscle testing or dowsing. For example, it is useful to know what the recommended intake of vitamin A is, or what the problem is with saturated fats, or the current thinking on the benefits of probiotics. This helps us to have a clarity when we test that may otherwise be missing. Yet it is important not to blindly accept current scientific and medical knowledge in this field. The history of science and medicine is a tale of many 'facts' being over-turned. So your testing may produce advice that does not appear to make sense in terms of current knowledge and your understanding of it. This could be, of course, because you have made a mistake in your testing and are coming to the wrong conclusions, but it can also be that the current scientific understanding is incorrect, or your own factual knowledge is limited in some way, or that this person is an exception to a generally accurate piece of nutritional knowledge.

I had a good example of this some years ago. I was doing a lot of allergy testing and finding many children allergic to artificial food colourings. I was delighted when natural food colourings were introduced by many manufacturers. But I was then totally taken aback when kinesiology testing showed that many children were allergic to the natural food colourings as well. This was not at all what I had expected or what had been suggested by advocates of natural food colouring. I often tested the food that the colouring was manufactured from (e.g. beetroot, tomato). Sometimes it would be a problem too, but sometimes it would be OK. This made no sense at all to me, but after careful retesting, I would go with what I had found. It was several years later that I began to understand about industrial solvents – chemicals that are used industrially to break down the cell walls of plants to extract the maximum amount of colour pigment from the plant. Then my findings with the children made sense – the ones that did not react to the fruit or vegetable source of the natural colouring must be reacting to minute traces of the solvent left behind by the industrial process. I was glad that I had stuck by what I had found even though it did not initially make sense.

Assessing Nutritional Advice

A report from Mintel, a UK market research company, found that 69% of 988 adults interviewed felt that it was hard to know which foods were healthy, because expert advice was always changing.

Of course, there are some nutritional recommendations that have stood the test of time and should be applied by everyone. Undoubtedly some people also use the changing expert advice to justify appalling eating habits on the grounds that nutritional advice is always changing so it is not worth following.

So, in the midst of all this we need some way of judging all this information and advice – from 'experts', the media, web sites, other therapists, books, etc., and deciding which is likely to have validity.

When I review nutritional information, advice and guidelines, I always review it in terms of the conditions that humankind have evolved in and the changes in the environment since then.

For example, people have survived well without nutritional supplements. Mankind has not evolved with a health store or pharmacy around the corner, so to argue that we all need to take supplements does not make sense from the viewpoint of mankind as hunter-gatherers.

It does make sense, however, if circumstances have changed so that life is now so different that supplementation is essential. This is the argument used for taking mineral supplements - the soil has become so depleted through constantly growing foods in the same ground that it no longer contains the nutrients for the plants, and so these are not available for us to access in this natural way.

Food combining (see page 103) does not make sense in terms of how we evolved. A hunter is unlikely to say, "I'm not eating these succulent berries that I have just come across because I've managed to slay and eat a deer an hour ago." (The protein in the deer is believed not to combine with fruit because of the different transit time in the gut for these different categories of food.) This does not mean that some people do not feel better when they food combine, but the fact that they do is an indication that they have some health problems. They may have digestive problems that need addressing, or food combining may have led them to exclude some allergen, or that by focussing on their diet they have realised what rubbish they eat and have stopped doing it. The fact that so many people benefit from food combining is an indication of how unhealthy many people are.

A common recommendation is that everyone should take fish oils, because they contain essential fatty acids (see page 80). 'Essential' means that the body needs them but cannot make them itself. So where does this leave vegetarians? Many people have evolved in places that do not have access to fish. There are two possibilities here. People with a genetic mutation that does not require these essential fatty acids have evolved in places where fish oils are not available. The alternative possibility is that there is a non-fish alternative source of essential fatty acids for those in areas with no access to fish. There are several alternatives such as pumpkin seeds and hemp oil. So, yes, an essential oil intake may be necessary for good health, but, no, it does not only have to come from fish.

For many years nutritionists talked about the importance of 'complete proteins'. Complete proteins contain all the essential amino acids that cannot be made by the human body. Amino acids (see page 73) are vitally important because they build enzymes, hormones, muscle, skin, hair, antibodies, etc. This was a particular issue for vegetarians because many of their sources of protein were not complete, unlike meat that has a full complement of the essential amino acids.

Vegetarians were urged to eat pulses and grains (e.g. baked beans on toast) at the same meal to ensure they achieved that magical complete protein. Scientists have now established that it is not necessary to eat all of them at the same time, as long as they are all eaten. This change in advice is hardly surprising for early man was an opportunistic hunter and forager and may have gone for long periods with no source of complete protein available.

I was listening recently to a radio interview with the author of a book on food cravings. She stated categorically that, after eating, insulin is produced which stops fat burning for 3 hours. She repeated this 'fact' several times, and from this had drawn various conclusions about what and how we should eat. One of the conclusions was that we should only eat three times a day – if we ate more frequently, then the insulin would stop our body burning fat. This information flies in the face of much practical research that suggests that eating frequent smaller meals containing some protein is the best way to reduce cravings and aid weight loss. This does not mean it is wrong – 'facts' do get regularly overturned, but this does not make sense on a lot of different levels. It is a very simple model of the body – hormones such as insulin interact with each other – and anyway there are huge differences between individuals. Also is the body really that precise? She did not say 'about 3 hours'. What happens if the person does something that demands a lot of calories in those three hours? It is difficult to believe that this theory will stand the test of time and be the miracle cure that she thinks.

In recent years there has been a lot of interest in antioxidants (see page 99), and some authorities urge everyone to take an antioxidant supplement. Antioxidants, which counter free-radical damage, are often labelled as the premier anti-ageing supplements, but does it make sense to say we need to take supplements? Excess free radical production can be caused by smoking, sunbathing, frying food, infections, excessive exercise, stress, radiation and environmental pollution. Exposure to the last three is certainly on the increase, and this could be sufficient in itself to support a recommendation for anti-oxidant supplementation. The fact that anti-oxidant supplementation is to counter ageing raises another issue. Evolution and selection is all about breeding. If you have the right gene variations that will allow you to live to a fertile age and breed more effectively, your genes are likely to have a good chance of surviving and becoming the norm. Gene variations that help us to live healthily into old age cannot be selected for in the same way, as it will not affect our ability to breed. Imagine a gene variation that means that women look as though they are 50 when they are 80 years old, with the women having 'normal levels' of fertility. This gene variation is less likely to be passed on than one that has 50-year-old women looking like 80-year-old women, but the women are highly fertile. Evolution does not select for variations that help us live healthily into old age, it selects for fecundity. Because of this, it is not illogical to think that we might need nutritional support to be healthy in old age.

There are a lot of books on the market that propose miracle solutions for health problems. Many of these seem to be of the type 'it worked for me so it will work for everyone with this problem'. These books are clearly genuine and enthusiastic attempts on the part of the author to spread good news and help people, but they do need to be looked at objectively.

Of course, there are also people with vested interests – nutritional supplement manufacturers, book authors, scientists, doctors, etc. – who, for their own reasons, may or may not want you to change what you eat and what supplements you take. But, this does not mean it is necessarily wrong. The reason I sell supplements is because I believe (and have seen the evidence) that people benefit from them.

So, when you are assessing nutritional knowledge bear in mind:

- It could be wrong, even if the book or the person giving the information sounds convincing.
- It could be wrong, even if the person giving the information believes totally that it is true.
- You could have misunderstood.
- It does not necessarily apply to everyone – we are all different.
- Does it make sense in terms of how we have evolved from being hunter-gatherers?
- Is it specifically aimed at improving people's post-fertile period of life?
- Does the person giving this knowledge have a vested interest in your believing it?

Ideal Diet

There is no such thing as the ideal diet that suits every body; just as people's appearances vary so their needs for food and nutrients vary. Each one of us is biologically individual. When working with clients, it is necessary to have a clear idea of what is mean by 'ideal diet'. Here is the definition I use:

The ideal diet for a person consists of:

the right food

in the right amounts

at the right time

in the right way

This ideal diet can vary over time. It is affected by changes in health, by therapy, by changes in life style and circumstances (e.g. age, stress, exercise, the contraceptive pill, recreational drugs), etc.

If the nutritional work forms a small part of a therapy session, it is usually appropriate to do the nutritional testing at the end, because the therapy work can change requirements. For example, if the session initiates a lot of healing, this could increase the client's need for vitamin C, zinc, etc. Your energy work may lead to metabolic changes, so that a supplement is no longer necessary. If you tested early in the session for the supplement, you might have to test all over again at the end of the session because the nutrient needs are now different.

Nutritional Indexes

Nutritional indexes can help in dietary analysis. A score of 100 on an index of 100 would indicate that no improvement could be made for that factor for that person. An index of 0 would mean it would not be possible to make it worse (although it may be possible to make it equally bad). **It is relatively easy to get most indexes up into the 80's, but the remaining increase can be much more difficult to achieve.**

When working out an index for the current situation it is important to have a time scale in mind, e.g. an index for the last week may be different to an index for the last year. Longer time scales are particularly appropriate if the person's life style and eating patterns are erratic.

Both insufficiency and excess will decrease a nutritional index.

The questioning might look like this:

> *On a scale of 0 to 100 where 100 is as good as it could be and 0 is as bad as it could be, what is Matthew's diet for the last three months? At least 50?* No
> *At least 40?* Yes
> *At least 45?* No
> [Etc.]

My book *Verbal Questioning Skills* has a lot more information on working with indexes.

If you are unhappy using a numerical scale then use the following descriptive index instead:

- **Disastrous** = actively creates illness
- **Very Poor** = stops a sick person getting well
- **Poor** = hampers recovery
- **Neutral** = no effect or benefits and problems cancel each other out
- **Good** = some deficiencies/excesses but generally O.K.
- **Very good** = no deficiencies/excesses
- **Excellent** = supports vibrant health

The questioning might look like this:

> *Looking at Matthew's diet for the last 3 months, has it been poor or worse?* Yes
> *Has it been poor?* No
> *Has it been very poor?* Yes

If the index is below 100 then there are four possibilities:

- Make changes to diet
- Introduce and/or make changes to one or more supplements
- Carry out energy work to enhance absorption etc.
- Advise on life style changes, e.g. giving up smoking, getting more rest.

It may be that you would look at more than one aspect. So, for example, you might work out dietary changes and do some energy work to help the person better digest raw food.

This book deals with only the first two options I any depth, but it is important when you are working to be aware of the other options.

Having established the index check in which areas work is needed and what is the priority order (see page 12).

Sometimes it is useful to ask what the index would be if the person did/did not do a particular thing, e.g. if the person gave up smoking, followed a specific exercise plan, ate more slowly, etc.

Testing for the time in the person's life at which a dietary index was highest can be useful, but be aware that the diet which was suitable then may not be suitable now (although in general there will be many factors in common). However, when you have established when the dietary index was at its highest, the client will often say something like: "Oh yes, I felt really good then. I had loads of energy and I didn't have all these spots." This puts the client in touch with how it feels to have a good (for them) diet, and can help motivate them to make the necessary changes now.

You can work with the nutrition session menu with or without using nutritional indexes.

Working With The Nutritional Menu

Most therapists offer other possibilities than just doing nutritional work, so how do you decide to work in this area?

1. Sometimes you will get clients (or friends and family) who say something like: "I've read this magazine article that says vitamin B is good for nerves. Do you think I should take some?" This is the simplest lead in to nutritional work, because you immediately have a question needing an answer.

2. Sometimes testing will suggest that nutrition is a key area for this person. You may have used dowsing or kinesiology to establish that what the client needs is some nutrition and diet advice. If you are a kinesiologist using finger modes, it could come up that way too.

The framework I usually use for nutritional work is the 'menu' (a particularly appropriate word in the circumstances) set out on pages 25 to 34. The menu lists all the possible things that can be checked (e.g. drinking more water, taking supplements, changing cooking utensils, using ritual, etc.)

This menu can be used in various ways:

1. Work out a full programme starting with the first item on the nutritional testing menu and work through it systematically.

2. Test for the priority from the nutritional testing menu.

3. Work out nutritional needs in relation to a specific problem, (e.g. weight loss, hay fever, diverticulitis, tiredness, dry skin, etc.) using the nutritional testing menu.

4. Work in relation to a specific piece of nutritional advice suggested by the client.

Working Out A Full Programme Starting At The Beginning Of The Menu

Work through the whole menu, checking each category as you go.

Although this may seem the most thorough approach, for many clients it will result in overload. If you give them too much to do, they may do nothing. You could get round this by limiting how much you find in any one session; e.g. you could find the first three things in one session and then carry on from where you left off in subsequent sessions.

Even if you do that, there is still a major problem with this approach: it could be that the really significant thing that is going to make the biggest changes may be towards the end of the menu, and you would not get to that very quickly.

For completeness I will give an example of how testing might look, but do bear in mind that you will very rarely, if ever, use this approach.

Would it be appropriate to do some questioning around method of eating? No
Would it be appropriate to do some work around temperature? No
Would it be appropriate to do some work around meals? No
Would it be appropriate to do some work around snacking? Yes
So, is it to increase snacking? No
To decrease snacking? Yes
[Etc.]

Testing For Priority

Test for the priority from the nutritional testing menu - work this up and then do further components if there is time and the body gives you energy permission.

Priority in this sense does not necessarily mean 'the most important thing to do'; it means 'the next thing to do'. Decide how much to do by carefully watching the client's response and by testing if you should establish more things to do, to take or to avoid.

For example, make a start and work out the first thing. If the client immediately said: "Oh, I can do that", test if you should add more and proceed in this way till you no longer have permission to add more, the client looks overloaded or you have run out of time. Once the client has fully incorporated those changes, you can add more changes at subsequent sessions.

We are looking for the priority item that the energy system wants working on using the concept of an ideal diet (see page 8).

Would it be appropriate to do some questioning around diet and supplements using the nutrition testing menu? Yes
Is the first thing we should look at on the first page? No
Is it on the second page? Yes
[Find the item on this page and work out the details]
Would it be appropriate to do more testing for the ideal diet now? Yes
Is the thing we are looking for on the first page? Yes
[Work out the item]
Would it be appropriate to do more testing for the ideal diet now? No
[You might want to ask when it would be appropriate to do more work in this area.]

This approach often works well combined with the use of nutritional indexes. As you work out each item, you can test what difference that will make to the person's current nutritional index (see page 9).

Nutrition Testing In Relation To A Specific Problem/Symptom
Use the nutritional menu, but base your questioning on a specific problem, e.g. asthma.

Clients that have been coming to see you for some time and trust you may be happy to make changes without knowing in detail what they are for. With new clients framing the work so that it is related to a specific symptom is often the best approach. New clients may not understand the rather global approach of working according to priority, and may not be committed enough at this early stage to accept working out a full nutritional programme either.

Symptoms are a way the body uses to tell us that something is wrong. Symptoms are signs that the body is unbalanced. If the body is using energy to produce symptoms, this is usually an indication that the underlying imbalance needs addressing soon if not immediately. In a way the testing is no different from the Testing Priority approach, except that the practitioner bears in mind that the work is in relation to a particular set of symptoms or named illness. It is good to keep reminding yourself that you are looking for help for a particular problem and not at the overall situation for the client. The easiest way to do this is to include the problem in the questioning rather than leaving it implied. Questioning might look like this:

> *Would it be appropriate to do some questioning around diet and supplements using the nutrition testing menu for Angela's diverticulitis?* Yes
> *Is the first thing we should look at for this problem on the first page?* No
> *Is it on the second page?* Yes
> [Find the item on this page and work out the details]
> *Would it be appropriate to do more testing for this problem now?* Yes
> Is it more nutritional work? Yes
> [Etc.]

Nutrition In Relation To Particular Advice/Information
Check if something the client wants to do would be appropriate.

Sometimes the client asks you to check some particular nutritional advice, e.g. "Do you think I should be taking any supplements?" or "I've read this book on food combining; do you think that would help me?" In the example here the client tells you that he has read that reducing fat intake is good for diverticulitis and wants to know if this would be good for him.

Would it be appropriate to do some work around fat consumption for James? Yes
Would changing fat consumption in some way have a positive effect on the diverticulitis?
Yes
Would it be appropriate to reduce fat intake? No
To change the type of fat in some way? Yes
[Etc.]

Notice the first question is slightly broader than the one asked by the client, as it does not specifically talk about reducing. This is deliberate – if you ask the question as the client framed it, the answer could be 'no', but a change in the proportion of different fats, for example, could be beneficial. As the client has raised this, he has some real interest in it, so it would be a shame to lose that by not framing the question broadly enough.

You could, of course, get that fat consumption should not be changed, but something else needs to be done.
e.g.:

Would it be appropriate to do some work around fat consumption for James? No
Are there any dietary changes that James could make that would help his diverticulitis?
Yes

[You are now into nutritional testing for a particular problem – see above.]

Another possibility is that making some changes around fat consumption is important for the client's health, but not in the way he thinks it might be. Questioning in that case might look like this:

Would it be appropriate to do some work around fat consumption for James? Yes
Would changing fat consumption in some way have a positive effect on the diverticulitis?
No
Would it have positive health benefits in other ways? Yes
{Work out what health area and what needs to be done]

I suggest you work out the health benefit before you work out what he needs to do. For example, changing his fat consumption in some way may help James' dry skin, but this may be a minor irritation compared with the diverticulitis. In this case it might be better to make a note to look at this area in a subsequent session once the diverticulitis problem is resolved.

Sometimes you might be the person who wants to check a piece of nutritional information. For example, you may have a client with psoriasis, and you have made some progress but not as much as you would like. You have now been sent some information on a new product that is supposed to be particularly good for psoriasis, and you want to ask specifically about this. In this case, you would turn to the part of the menu that deals with supplements (page 132), but the exact part of the menu would vary according to the nature of the advice you want to test.

General Consideration And The Nutrition Session Menu

The nutritional session menu (pages 25 to 34) is the heart of this book. It may look rather daunting and complicated, but once you learn to use it you will find you quickly can home in on what elements about the client's diet and nutrition need changing and what those changes should be. You can see an example of how it is used in Appendix F.

When I first started using kinesiology for nutritional testing I had a very simple menu with 4 basic questions – does the person need to:

- Start something?
- Increase something?
- Stop something?
- Decrease something?

But I rapidly realised this was inadequate. For example, if I found that the person needed to increase something, I realised this could be an individual food (e.g. apples), a nutrient (e.g. foods high in vitamin C), a group of foods (e.g. all fruit), etc.

Making matters even more complicated I realised that this increase might be only at a particular time of the day (e.g. at 3.00pm or before noon) or connected to a particular activity (e.g. immediately after exercise).

What had started as a simple 4-question procedure was mushrooming out of control, and I became nervous of venturing into this area. It all seemed too complicated. But I knew that nutrition and diet are vitally important to people's long-term health, and so this menu started to evolve over several years.

As I worked with the menu, I realised that there were some general considerations that applied across the whole field, so you always need to bear the following in mind when you are working with the nutritional menu.

Setting Things Up

You can set up muscle testing or dowsing to respond in a certain way. For example, in muscle testing you could set up the 'yes' response to be a weak/unlocked response from the muscle, and the 'no' response to be a strong/locked response. The important point is not what you do, but that you do it consistently, so you can reliably interpret what the muscle response means. Occasionally

I have had students test a muscle, get a response and then say to me: "What does that mean?" Before you do any testing, you should be completely clear what the different responses mean. Otherwise you are unlikely to get meaningful testing results.

Knock-On Effects

Making changes in one area may mean that changes need to be made elsewhere. For example, if you test that the person needs to increase their fibre intake, they will probably also need to increase their water intake. It is possible to find this in two ways.

Firstly, you could find it by asking:

> *Is there anything else we need to know about this?*

And then, when you get the answer 'yes', you test till you find that the person needs to increase their water intake.

The other way is for it to come up by getting 'no' to

> *Is there anything else we need to know about this?*

Then 'yes' to

> *Is there something else we need to do'*

And then you test on the menu till you get to 'water'.

The advantage of the first option is that it is totally clear that the two are connected. The advantage of the second option is that in practice it often makes the questioning more manageable. In general I use the second method, but you can set it up either way. Just be consistent about which you do. By 'set it up' I mean you are very clear about what the implication of an answer 'yes' would be, and that you are consistent in this clarity.

The Logic Of Order

Sometimes you need to establish several things about an item. For example, if you establish from the menu that you are looking for the timing of drinking water in relation to meals, you need to know which meal or meals, and also what the time interval is, and whether it is before or after the meal(s).

It is easy to focus on the timing aspect first, as this is after all what it is named on the menu. But it is important to establish which meal (or meals) you are talking about first, because it could be one specific meal (e.g. no water for one hour before dinner) or it could be several meals or even all meals (e.g. drink a large glass of water with lunch and dinner).

Here is an example of how <u>not</u> to do it:

> *Am I looking at drinking water in relation to meals?* Yes
> *Is it before the meal?*

The questioner has assumed that the information is about one meal only, (but even then it would be logical to establish <u>which</u> meal first). On paper this error may look obvious, but this was a very common error of course participants when I taught nutritional testing as a workshop. Here is an example of a correct way of doing it – there are other ways too:

> *Am I looking at drinking water in relation to meals?* Yes
> *Is it in relation to all meals?* Yes
> *Is it the same information for all the meals?* No
> *Are there restrictions/requirements for all the meals?* No
> *Are there restrictions/requirements for breakfast?* Yes
> *For lunch?* No
> *For the evening meal?* Yes
> *OK, so for breakfast ....*

Having got the information about breakfast, you would then need to ask about the evening meal but (in this case) not about lunch.

Finding A Specific Food Or A Specific Food Category

Quite often you will need to establish a particular food or food category. This may be to avoid or to eat more of, to eat at a particular time of day or avoid at a particular time of day, and so on. Firstly you need to establish whether you are looking for a particular food or a category of food:

> *Am I looking for a food category?* No
> *Am I looking for a particular food?* Yes

Regardless of whether you are looking for a category of food (e.g. meat or foods rich in vitamin C or foods in the deadly nightshade family) or looking for an individual item (e.g. carrots or plaice or hamburgers) start with the classifications.

I use 3 different ways of classifying foods:

1) Culinary Classification – see Appendix BI
2) Nutritional Classification – see Appendix B2
3) Botanical Food Families – see Appendix B3

Note that these are different ways of classifying the same things, so all simple foods appear in all three categories. For example, you could find carrot via 'culinary' classification (vegetables), via 'nutritional classification (foods rich in beta carotene) and via 'botanical' classification (parsley family).

If you are looking for a category, you stop earlier in the questioning process than if you are looking for the individual item. First you establish which type of classification to use – culinary, nutritional or botanical. Then you find the category within that classification, e.g.

> *Which would be the <u>most</u> appropriate way to categorise the food – in terms of culinary classification?* Yes

When you ask for the most appropriate way, you are in a sense asking for the easiest and quickest way. The botanical list is particularly useful for some of the less obvious things (e.g. buckwheat). The culinary categories are often useful for finding more complex foods (e.g. the burger the client eats from time to time).

Establishing A Food Category

Having established the best way to find the food category, you then start asking detailed questions. So, for example, having established that you are looking for a group within the culinary classification (see appendix B1), you then ask:

> *Is it meat?* No
> *Is it fish?* Yes

Remember that you are looking for a <u>category</u> of food, not a specific food, so you do not find a specific fish, although you could be looking for a sub-category within fish, e.g.

> *Is it all fish?* No
> *Is it shellfish?* Yes
> *Just shellfish?* Yes

Establishing A Specific Food

When finding a specific food you can use the food categories to help narrow down the options, e.g.

> *Which type of classification would help me find the food most quickly – is it the culinary classification?* Yes
> *Is it a meat?* No
> *Is it a fish?* No
> *Is it a dairy product?* Yes [Note it cannot be all dairy on this occasion because you are looking for a specific food rather than a whole category].
> *Is it milk?* No
> *Is it cheese?* Yes
> *A specific cheese?* No

Another way of narrowing down the options is to ask when the client commonly eats the food, e.g.

Is the food we are looking for normally eaten at most meals? No
Is the food eaten at one or more specific meals? No
Is it usually eaten between meals? Yes [Consult client to find out the sort of things eaten between meals.]
Is it any of the things the client has mentioned? No [Consult client again, who then remembers that she has a packet of chewing gum that she keeps in the car and chews while driving.]
Is it the chewing gum? Yes
Is it all chewing gum? Yes

Detrimental Foods

When working with detrimental foods/drinks (e.g. alcohol, processed food etc.), you are normally asking about the <u>maximum</u> amount not the optimum amount. You need to be clear in how you give your client this information: you are not saying they must have x bars of chocolate a week; you are telling them that 'x' is the maximum they can consume without causing lasting damage to their health. Emphasise this, because otherwise you will get people eating that amount of chocolate even though it is not beneficial. I usually say something like: "Testing says you can eat a maximum of two bars of chocolate a week without long term damage to your health. That doesn't mean you should do this, as it is not giving you any benefit."

Beneficial Foods

When working with beneficial food/drink (e.g. organic food, good water, etc.) then you are normally asking about the <u>optimum</u> or in some situations you may be asking about the <u>minimum</u> amount.

- Minimum – if people are short of money or reluctant to do something you might want to ask for the minimum for the person to receive any benefit.

- Optimum – what will give the most benefit either in general or for a particular problem

Avoidance, Replacements, Reductions And Additions

Sometimes a client will need to avoid a substance completely, either indefinitely or for a period of time. Some years ago I had a client who was severely allergic to fish: his throat would begin to close up with even the smallest amount of fish stock. I carried out various energy procedures to correct this, but testing then showed that it would take six months before he could eat any fish without reacting. I tested how much he could eat that first time and it was a very small quantity. I tested how long he must wait before he ate more fish and how much it should be. It took quite a while to work out an extremely detailed programme for his fish intake, but testing showed that he would eventually be able to eat several varieties of fish in normal quantities. When I saw him again many months later, he told me that he had followed my instructions to the letter and was now eating fish without any problem.

Normally it is not necessary to work out such a detailed programme as this for the reintroduction of a food. In general having established when the client can first eat the food, I then check if I need to establish more detailed information (e.g. how much, how soon can increase from that, etc.). Very often this is not necessary. Presumably it was in this case because of the client's extreme reaction.

When you test that someone needs to decrease or exclude something, it is important to look at what they might do instead. For example, if you test that the client should reduce the amount of coffee they drink, you need to ask them out loud what they would like to replace it with and then test if that is an appropriate substitute. Otherwise they could follow your instruction and drink less coffee, but replace it with black tea or chamomile tea, which are allergens for them. E.g. you have found out that the client, who normally drinks seven cups of coffee a day, should drink a maximum of two. When you ask her what she would drink instead, she says: "Probably tea, or may be that new orange drink I saw advertised on the TV." Check how she would drink her tea (with milk, sugar etc.) and the orange drink (with ice, a lemon slice, etc.) You then start testing:

> *Would it cause any harm to Lily if she drank 5 cups of tea with sweetener a day to replace the coffee she drinks now?* Yes
> *So is it appropriate for any of the substitute to be tea as she's described it?* No
> *If she left out the sweetener, would it then be suitable?* Yes
> [Cry of dismay from the client and "Well, I'd have to have sugar then"]
> *So, if she added a teaspoonful of sugar instead, would this be suitable?* Yes
> Would it be appropriate for all 5 cups to be tea like this? No
> [Find the number and then check the orange drink.]

If the person needs to increase something, the same considerations apply. For example, if the client needs to increase fruit intake, ask them what specific fruits they would choose to add and then check that this selection is appropriate.

Banking Food

When an item is being restricted, the concept of 'banking' food is useful. For example, you might work out that a client can tolerate 100 grams of chocolate a day, or a quarter of a cup of coffee a day. On being told this, the client may well ask if it is possible to save this up and have it all at one time. I developed the concept of 'banking food' in response to this sort of question. I have found that the easiest way to phrase a question to answer this type of query from a client is to ask:

> *How many days would it be appropriate for you to bank food – at least three?* No
> *At least two?* Yes
> *So, Emma can have 200 grams of chocolate every other day, or 100 grams every day, is that correct?* Yes

Note that what this means is that the client can never bank more than two days' chocolate. So, for example, if Emma had not had any chocolate for three days she could still only have 200 grams, because that is the maximum amount she is allowed to 'save'.

In the coffee example, you might test that they can bank up to 5 days' worth of coffee. You would then explain to the client that they can have a quarter of a cup of coffee a day, or save it up and have half a cup every two days, or a full cup every four days, or a cup and a quarter every five days. They can vary what they do, but they cannot 'save' the coffee for longer than five days or 'draw out' any more than what they have saved at any particular time.

What Happens Then?
It is important not to assume that when the time is over the activity stops. The activity could:

- Increase (e.g. a larger dose of a supplement, more frequent meals, etc.).
- Reduce (e.g. take 2 capsules instead of 3, etc.).
- Stop.
- Change in some way (e.g. supplement now taken at a different time of the day).
- Alternate (e.g. take a different type of calcium for three weeks, then back to the original one for four weeks and so on).

If the activity is continuing till the next appointment, you can check out during that appointment what should happen next. If the person is not coming back for another appointment, or the appointment date is after the final date for the activity, you need to check at the time what happens after this date. The questioning might look like this:

So, do we increase the supplement? No
Reduce it? No
Stop? No
Change it in some way? Yes
Type of supplement? No
When taken? Yes
[Etc.]

How Precise Do You Need To Be?

It is difficult to give blanket guidance on precision, because situations vary so much. It is easy to feel you always have to be absolutely precise, but in reality too much precision can be unhelpful.

For example, you might be testing the timing for lunch (see page 40); you could test down to the precise minute (or even the nanosecond), but is that really necessary or beneficial? You might test that the client should eat lunch at 1.06, but what happens if the client eats lunch at 1.07? You can easily imagine an anxious client getting very stressed, because it's now 1.10, and he has not started eating yet. This is not going to improve his digestion when he does eat his meal.

Common sense often will suggest how precise you need to be, but do confirm this with testing. Here is an example where you have already narrowed the time down somewhat:

> *So, James needs to eat his lunch between 1 and 1.30, is that correct?* Yes
> *Do we need to be more precise?* Yes
> Between 1.00 and 1.15? Yes
> *Do we need to be more precise?* No

Client Imagines The Scenario

For some types of behavioural change it can be quite difficult to describe accurately in words what the client needs to do. If you find yourself struggling in this way, one possibility might be to ask the client to visualise doing the action (e.g. chewing in a particular way) and then you test if the way it is being visualised is correct. You work in this way with the client till they have the correct visualising. It is important that these visualisations are really vivid, as the clients need to retain the images long after they have left your office.

Clients Helping Out

Sometimes the client will try to 'help out' in the questioning by saying: "Oh, I know what this is … it's …" Sometimes they are right, but no matter how plausible what they say sounds it is important to check it out. Here is an example:

> *Is what John has suggested correct?* No
> *Is it along the right lines?* Yes
> *OK, so John suggested this was about how he misses breakfast and just has lots of coffee.*
> *Is that what we should be looking at?* No
> *Is this about his coffee consumption?* Yes
> *Throughout the day?* Yes
> [Etc.]

Looking At All the Options

At various places in the menu you will see the word 'other'. This is an important category, as it allows you to find things that are not already listed. You will need to ask systematic questions to find what it is you are looking for. (See my book *Verbal Questioning Skills For Kinesiologists*.)

In the menu you will also see some items with brackets round them {xxx}. This means that this option is unlikely given our current understanding of nutrition, but is included for completeness.

Confirmation

Throughout the testing it is important to ask questions that are a confirmation. There are two ways I usually use to do this:

- Asking an opposing question
- Asking a summarising question.

Opposing questions are where you rephrase the question in a way that means you would expect the opposite muscle or pendulum response, e.g.

> *Is it 8 glasses of water a day?* Yes
> *Is it more than 8?* No

Summarising questions are particularly useful when what you have found so far is very complicated, e.g.

> *Sam has to drink 8 glasses of water a day in addition to what he is already drinking. At least two of those glasses should be with breakfast, and he shouldn't drink any water with lunch. Is that correct?*

If you got that the summarising question was incorrect, you would break it down to find out which bit was incorrect, e.g.

> *Is it correct that Sam has to drink 8 glasses of water a day in addition to what he is already drinking?* Yes
> *Is it correct that at least two of these glasses should be with breakfast?* No
> *Is it the quantity that is incorrect for the breakfast water?* No
> *Is it the timing?* Yes
> *So, should it be before breakfast?* Yes
> *Do I need to establish how much before?* Yes
> [And so on …]

Once you have this bit correct, you would go back to your original summarising question, make the changes and ask it again.

It is vitally important that these confirmation questions are tested with due care and attention. Do not just go through the motions, assuming you have got it correct. It can seem tedious, but what is the point of saving time but giving clients inaccurate information?

The Nutritional Testing Menu

04 Snacking *page 50*
- ➢ Increase
- ➢ Decrease
- ➢ Specific foods

05 Timing *page 49*
- ➢ Meals *page 49*
  - ∗ All meals
  - ∗ One specific meal
- ➢ Earliest/latest time to eat *page 50*
- ➢ Category of food
- ➢ One specific food
- ➢ Supplement(s) *Appendix D2*
- ➢ Drugs *Appendix D2*
- ➢ Other

06 Food Quality *page 52*
- ➢ Organic *page 52*
- ➢ Freshness
- ➢ Other

07 Food Storage and Preparation *page 54*
- ➢ Temperature of storage *page 54*
  - ∗ Fridge
  - ∗ Freezer
  - ∗ Particular food or category
- ➢ Light/Dark *page 55*
- ➢ Containers, Wrappers And Utensils *page 55*
  - ∗ Phthalates
  - ∗ Aluminium
  - ∗ Nickel
  - ∗ Lead
  - ∗ Iron
  - ∗ Clay
  - ∗ Other

➢ Method of cooking
  ∗   Microwave cooking *page 56*
  ∗   Frying *page 56*
  ∗   Other
➢ Other

08   **Total Calories** *page 59*
  ➢ Calories
   ∗   Decrease
   ∗   Increase
  ➢ Exercise (outside the scope of this book)

09   **Carbohydrate And The Glycaemic Index** *page 62*
  ➢ Increase carbohydrate generally
  ➢ Decrease carbohydrate generally
  ➢ Increase low glycaemic index foods
   ∗   Specific food(s)
   ∗   In general
   ∗   Time of day
   ∗   Activity related
  ➢ Decrease low glycaemic index foods
   ∗   As above
  ➢ Increase high glycaemic index foods
   ∗   As above
  ➢ Decrease high glycaemic index foods
   ∗   As above

10   **Water** *page 65*
  ➢ Quantity
   ∗   In relation to meals
   ∗   In relation to a food category
   ∗   In relation to a specific food
   ∗   In relation to an activity
   ∗   Other
  ➢ Quality
  ➢ Timing *page 40*
  ➢ Other

11 Fibre *page 69*
  - Soluble
    - * Increase
    - * {Decrease} - **unlikely**
  - Insoluble
    - * Increase
    - * Decrease

12 Protein *page 71*
  - Overall quantity
    - * Increase
    - * Reduce
  - Particular type of protein
    - * Increase
    - * Reduce
  - Particular amino acid *page 73*
    - * Increase
    - * Reduce
  - Timing *page 40*

13 Oils And Fats *page 79*
  - Saturated fats *page 82*
    - * Increase in general
    - * Increase specific ones
    - * Decrease in general
    - * Decrease specific one(s)
  - Polyunsaturated fats *page 82*
    - * Increase in general
    - * Increase specific one(s)
    - * Decrease in general
    - * Decrease specific one(s)
  - Monounsaturated fats *page 82*
    - * Increase in general
    - * Increase specific one(s)
    - * Decrease in general
    - * Decrease specific one(s)
  - Transfatty acids *page 83*
    - * {Increase in general} - **unlikely**
    - * {Increase specific one(s)} - **unlikely**

16 Minerals *page 94* and *Appendix A2*
- ➢ Increase
  - * Through food
  - * Through supplements *page 132*
- ➢ Decrease
  - * Through food
  - * Through supplements *page 132*

17 Phytochemicals *page 96*
- ➢ Increase
  - * In general
  - * Specific food(s)
  - * Supplements *page 132*
- ➢ {Decrease} - **unlikely**
  - * See under increase phytochemicals

18 Antioxidants *page 98*
- ➢ Increase
  - * In general
  - * Foods
    - − Anti-oxidant groups *page 99*
    - − Specific food
  - * Supplements *page 132*
- ➢ {Decrease} - **unlikely**
  - * As under increase

19 Prebiotics And Probiotics *page 101*
- ➢ Increase prebiotics
  - * Food
  - * Supplement *page 132*
- ➢ Decrease prebiotics
  - * Food
  - * Supplement *page 132*
- ➢ Increase Probiotics
  - * Food
  - * Supplement *page 132*

➤ Decrease Probiotics
  * Food
  * Supplement *page 132*

20 Food Combining / Uncombining *page 103*
  ➤ Standard food combining advice
  ➤ Standard food combining advice with variations
  ➤ Combining foods *page 17*
    * Food category with food category
    * Specific food with particular food
    * Specific food with a category of food
  ➤ Uncombining foods
    * As above
  ➤ Other

21 Acid Alkaline Balance *page 107*
  ➤ {Decreasing alkaline forming foods} **- unlikely**
  ➤ Decreasing acid forming foods
    * Overall
    * Particular food type *page 17*
  ➤ Increasing alkaline forming foods
    * Overall
    * Particular food type *page 17*
  ➤ {Increasing acid forming foods} **- unlikely**

22 Raw/ Cooked Foods *page 110*
  ➤ Decreasing raw foods *page 17*
    * All
    * Category of foods
    * Specific food (s)
  ➤ Increasing raw food
    * As above
  ➤ Decreasing cooked foods
    * As above
  ➤ Increasing cooked food
    * As above

23 Processed Foods *page 112*
> ➤ Decrease processed food *page 17*
>> * Group of foods
>> * Specific food
> ➤ {Increase} processed food - **unlikely**

24 Food Additives *page 114*
> ➤ Decrease/stop food additive(s)
>> * Individual additive
>> * Particular category
> ➤ {Increase food additives} - **unlikely**

25 Stimulants And Anti-Nutrients *page 116*
> ➤ Alcohol *page 116*
>> * Decrease
>> * {Increase} - **unlikely**
> ➤ Caffeine *page 117*
>> * Decrease
>> * {Increase} - **unlikely**
> ➤ Tea *page 118*
>> * Decrease
>> * {Increase} - **unlikely**
> ➤ Coffee *page 118*
>> * Decrease
>> * {Increase} - **unlikely**
> ➤ Sugar *page 119*
>> * Decrease
>> * {Increase} - **unlikely**
> ➤ Artificial Sweeteners *page 119*
>> * Decrease
>> * {Increase} - **unlikely**

26 Allergy *page 120*
> ➤ Food category *page 17 and Appendix B1 to B3*
>> * Energy work (outside the scope of this book)
>> * Avoid
> ➤ Specific food
>> * As above

- ➤ Drink
  - ✻ As above
- ➤ Nutritional supplements *page 132*
  - ✻ As above
- ➤ Incidentals
  - ✻ As above

27 Tolerance *page 123*
- ➤ Food category *page 17 and Appendix B1 to B3*
  - ✻ Energy work (outside the scope of this book)
  - ✻ Avoid
- ➤ Specific food
  - ✻ As above
- ➤ Drink
  - ✻ As above
- ➤ Nutritional supplements *page 132*
  - ✻ As above
- ➤ Incidentals
- ➤ As above

28 Vital Energy *page 126*
- ➤ Avoid /Decrease
  - ✻ Food *page 17*
  - ✻ Drink
  - ✻ Nutritional supplements *page 132*
  - ✻ Incidentals
- ➤ Start/Increase
  - ✻ Food *page 17*
  - ✻ Drink
  - ✻ Nutritional supplements *page 132*
  - ✻ Incidentals

29 Specific Dietary Programme *page 128*
- ➤ Vegetarian *page 128*
- ➤ Vegan *page 129*
- ➤ Macrobiotic *page 129*
- ➤ Blood Group Diet *page 130*
- ➤ Atkins Diet *page 197*
- ➤ Other

30 Supplements *Page 132* and *Appendix A1 and A2*
- ➤ Check existing supplements
  - ✳ Beneficial and optimal
  - ✳ Beneficial but not optimal
  - ✳ Beneficial but something about it needs to be changed
  - ✳ Harmful
  - ✳ Neither beneficial or harmful
- ➤ New Supplements
  - ✳ Specific Manufacturer
  - ✳ Vitamins *page 90* and *Appendix A1*
  - ✳ Minerals *page 94* and *Appendix A2*
  - ✳ Amino Acid *page 73*
  - ✳ Oils *page 79*
  - ✳ Antioxidants *page 99*
  - ✳ Prebiotics And Probiotics *page 101*
  - ✳ Other

31 Other

This category allows you to find information and advice that cannot be accessed through any other part of the menu.

{ } = this is an unlikely category that the body would want, but for the sake of completeness it is included in the menu

What Are The Outcomes?

Getting clients to make and keep changes can be difficult. One way you can motivate them is by testing what will happen if they make the changes shown by testing. Even when you are working directly with the nutrition menu in terms of a particular symptom, there may be other benefits which are worth knowing about in order to increase client motivation to carry out the necessary changes.

It is important to decide on a time scale before starting, because, for example, there may be no noticeable change for 2 weeks, and then improvements will become evident. The easiest way to do this is to start with an arbitrary time and ask if the person will notice any changes. If you get a negative answer to this, move to a longer time period until you get a positive response. In general I do not worry about being very precise on this – I do not worry if the improvement will be in 20 days or 21 days – three weeks is an adequate guide here.

In addition it is important in the testing to be clear that you are asking about the client <u>noticing</u> changes. This is important because changes can be happening in the body but with no observable result. In this situation if you just asked about improvements you could get 'yes' even though the client would be totally unaware, and so the testing would appear to be wrong. Also some clients do not seem to notice any improvement unless their symptoms have completely disappeared. I remember a client of mine who came back looking a lot better but saying his eczema was no better. I checked his notes where I had listed all the areas of the body covered by the eczema and pointed out to him that he now only had eczema on one part of his body. He then conceded that his eczema was better. To cover all this use the person's name in the questioning, e.g. when will John notice the difference.

Here are some possibilities when testing for improvements, but this list is not comprehensive:

- Existing symptoms that the client has told you about, i.e. information you have listed on the client notes.

- Existing symptoms you do not know about – symptoms the client forgot to tell you about or assumed could not be fixed so did not mention.

- Physical body system (e.g. immune system, digestive system, etc.)

- Physical body part or parts. (e.g. joints less stiff – this would only come up here, if the client were unaware of this as a symptom. This happens remarkably often, because a particular problem has developed over time or has always been with them.)

- Other body functions, e.g. easier breathing, greater ability to resist infection, etc.

- Weight (e.g. weight gain, weight loss, redistribution of fat).

- Other physical appearance improvements (e.g. glossier hair, stronger nails).

- Physical energy levels (e.g. overall increase, more stable energy levels, increase at a particular time of day / associated with an activity, etc.).

- Allergy / tolerance and addictive behaviour (e.g. able to eat more wheat without experiencing problems, easier to resist cigarettes, etc.)

- Strength / flexibility.

- Pain (e.g. less frequent, less severe, etc.)

- Sleep (e.g. easier to get to sleep, wake more refreshed, less disturbed during night, etc.)

- Sex (e.g. increased sexual libido, more satisfaction, increased sensitivity, easier / more reliable orgasms, etc.)

- Emotional symptoms (e.g. improvement in ability to control emotions in general or a specific emotion, higher levels of positive emotions in general or a specific emotion, fewer mood swings, greater self-confidence, higher self-esteem, etc.)

- Mental symptoms (e.g. improved memory, greater alertness, better concentration, etc.)

- Performance (e.g. improved performance in general, in work, in sport, etc.)

Of course, one possibility is that the improvement would be in stopping something happening in the future, i.e. preventive. The client is likely to be unaware of this, but I still usually test for this specifically too.

Testing might look like this:

> *If John implemented the three changes we have worked out today, would he experience some noticeable benefit within two weeks?* No
> *If John implemented the three changes we have worked out today, would he experience some noticeable benefit within a month?* Yes
> *Would it be or include one of the symptoms we have in his case notes?* Yes
> *Is it the constant tiredness?* Yes
> [Get more detail if appropriate]
> Any of the other symptoms we have listed in the case notes? No
> Anything else? Yes
> *A symptom I don't know about?* No
> A change to a body system? Yes
> [Etc.]

Sometimes it is more appropriate to test what will happen if they do not make the changes, so what the penalties are. For example, if the client does not make the changes, the migraines will probably get worse, or they will probably start to experience a lot of colds and infections. Testing is very similar to for the benefits.

Testing about the future can be fraught because you do not know what other changes may occur in the client's life, so your testing is always a projection rather than a prediction. For this reason it is generally easier to be accurate about the next few weeks rather than the next few years.

Meaningful Instructions

It is extremely important that you give people meaningful instructions and measurements. Occasionally I meet people who have been given some instruction by their practitioner that they did not understand, e.g. eat 90 grams of protein a day. How can the client carry out an instruction they do not understand? A lot of people particularly have problems with measurements, so I often ask them how they would like me to measure.

So for example, if you test that someone needs to drink more water, you should first ask the client if they want you to check the total amount they should have each day, or the additional amount they should add to what they are already drinking. Both of these measurement methods will get you to the same result in terms of the amount the person should drink, but people tend to vary in which method they find easiest to apply.

Then, before you do any quantity testing, you ask the client what measurements to use. Possibilities (in the UK at least) include litres, pints, fluid ounces, mugfuls, cupfuls, and glassfuls. If you were measuring food, you'd be able to measure in handfuls, ounces, grams, slices, portions (as long as you are clear how big a 'portion' is), etc.

If the client wants to measure in terms of glasses, you ask them to indicate with their hands how big the glass is, and for them to keep that glass in mind while you muscle test how many glasses. I put this particular bit of the procedure in place after I tested someone for how many mugs of tea he could drink, only to find out later he had a mug at home that was half a litre and this was the mug he had in mind, while I had a much smaller mug in mind. Lack of clarity like this can lead to confusion and inaccurate testing.

At first sight this can all appear very complicated, but once you have done it a few times it becomes much easier.

Before you get in to measuring anything spend some time weighing and measuring lots of different foods and drinks in all the different units that people are likely to want you to measure in. E.g. see what a handful of grapes looks like, now weigh it. Pour out a glass of water, then put it into a measuring jug and see what the volume is.

When you have completed all the testing, write down your recommendations clearly, giving a copy to the client and keeping one yourself. Ask clients to read through the recommendations themselves, and then check that they understand everything. This is best done by asking them: "Do you have any questions about what I have written?"

Quantity And Timing

Quantity and timing questions can appear in lots of different situations when working with nutrition. Here is an overview of the most common possibilities.

How Much?

You may want to know how many tablets a person needs to take. Or how much of a food the person can tolerate.

You first have to decide on the units of measurement:

Supplements - this is usually easy as it will be the number of tablets/capsules/measures.

Food etc. - you have to decide first how to measure. Use some unit that is meaningful to the client. Give the client various options and ask if they have a preference, e.g. would they prefer ounces, grams or spoonfuls? If they would prefer spoonfuls what size spoon would they prefer?. For some things you might want to use the measure "normal portion" or "typical slice of bread" or "my favourite mug". If you are doing this, ask the client to indicate with their hands how big this is before you start doing the questioning. For extra reliability you can also ask them to imagine the measure as you do the testing.

The fastest way to establish the exact number is to ask in one of the following ways:

At least X:
If you ask *Is it at least 4?* and get the answer "yes", then the number is 4, 5, 6 , 7, etc.

X or more:
This is the same as "at least X"

More than X:
If you ask *Is it more than 4?* and get the answer "yes" , then the number is <u>not</u> 4 , but would be 5,6,7,etc.

Less than X:
If you ask *Is it less than 4?* and get the answer "yes", then the number is 0,1,2 0r 3

It is important to choose <u>one</u> of these methods and stick to it.

Once you have asked this first question, you can narrow it down with further questioning. See my book *Verbal Questioning Skills For Kinesiologists* for more information on this.

Clock Time

The most obvious way to work with time is in either clock time (e.g. at 4.30 pm or every 2 hours) or calendar time (on January 19th, every Wednesday).

For clock time you first need to establish your unit of measurement. It could be seconds, hours, days, months, a precise date or time, or indefinitely. Sometimes the context you are working in will narrow down the possible choices. For example, if you have established that a client with a severe infection needs to take vitamin C, you might well be working in hours, e.g. the client takes the vitamin C supplement every two hours for the rest of the day.

If you were determining when the client should change something in the future (e.g. their supplement regime), you would probably be asking for a specific date, e.g. June 25th. Often from a practical point of view a precise date is more useful than a time-span. For example, if you tested that a client should stop taking a particular supplement in 4 weeks, the client then has to work out what date that would be, so it is much better in these situations to work in terms of a date from the start. Here is an example of how this might look:

> *Is this supplement taken indefinitely?* No
> *Is it taken for the rest of this month?* No
> *At least until the 20th of this month?* Yes
> *At least until the 25th of this month?* No
> [Continue till you work out the exact date.]

When you are establishing time, you will sometimes be looking for a time-window, that is a period of time rather than a precise time. E.g. the person needs to eat their lunch sometime between noon and 1.25 pm. In this case you are looking for two times.

How long is indefinitely? In conventional terms indefinitely is a long, long time. In testing terms I usually limit it to 6 months. So, if the client tests to take a supplement indefinitely, I usually explain to them that this is a guide (as situations can change) and that after 6 months the situation should be reassessed even if everything has gone smoothly.

Clock Time Versus Activity Time

I used to assume that whenever I was asking about timing (how long for or how often) I would be working according to clock time or calendar time, e.g. until December 20th, at 6.30 p.m., three times a day, every other day, etc. Then one day I was working with a client and had a lot of difficulty establishing when she needed to do something. After a lot of head scratching I realised that there was the possibility of activity time, so that something is done in relation to another activity.

So now whenever I am faced with a time question, I first ask:

Are we measuring in clock time?

If I get 'no' to this, I ask:

Are we measuring in activity time?

Activity Time
There are three basic options for activity time:

- *Is this until some activity stops?*
  e.g. until the client stops smoking, until the client stops living in that place.

- *Is this until some activity starts?*
  e.g. until the client buys a particular supplement or until the next session.

- *Or, is this when some activity happens?*
  e.g. bedtime, or half an hour before breakfast, or every time the client menstruates.

For nutritional questioning the most obvious possibilities are in relation to getting up, going to bed or eating meals. Here is an example where you are establishing when a person needs to drink an extra glass of water:

So, are we measuring in clock time? No
In activity time? Yes
Is this in relation to a meal or meals? Yes
Is it all meals? Yes
And is the timing the same in relation to all meals? Yes
So is it at the same time as the meal? No
Before the meal? Yes
Immediately before? No
So, are we looking for a time window here? Yes
Is the latest time at least 10 minutes? Yes
Do I need to be more exact? No
Is the earliest time at most 30 minutes before the meal? No
Is the earliest time at most 20 minutes before the meal? Yes
Do I need to be more exact? No
OK, so the water should be drunk 10 to 20 minutes before each meal. Is that correct?
Yes

There are other activity times that do not link to being awake or meals. Here are some activity time examples to give you a clearer idea of the possibilities:

- Take the supplement whenever you don't rest for at least half an hour during the afternoon.

- Avoid wheat whenever you have oranges or orange juice in the day.

- Take the supplement when you work for more than 8 hours in a day.

- Take the supplement when you feel you are about to lose your temper.

- Drink a litre of water half an hour before you start a gym workout.

- Double you intake of the zinc supplement whenever you can feel your eczema about to break out again.

- Don't eat chocolate on days you visit your mother.

- Avoid all dairy until the next appointment.

- Take the supplement until all your symptoms have been clear for at least two weeks.

- Take the supplements until you give up smoking.

- Don't eat wheat until you can flex your wrists without pain.

Of course, these are just examples and the actual possibilities are endless.

Method Of Eating (01)

On the menu we have:

01 Method of Eating
- ➢ Chewing
    - ＊ Chewing each mouthful
    - ＊ Time between mouthfuls
- ➢ Sipping
    - ＊ All liquids
    - ＊ Liquids at a particular temperature
    - ＊ A particular liquid
- ➢ Smelling/tasting/touching
- ➢ Eating with conscious awareness
- ➢ Setting and ritual
- ➢ Body position
- ➢ Other

Chewing

Chewing is important for digestion (particularly carbohydrates) because:

- It breaks down the food so that when it reaches the stomach the stomach juices can interact with it more quickly.

- Saliva contains an enzyme ptyalin (also called salivary amylase) that changes carbohydrates into maltose and dextrin.

- The water in the saliva starts the process of dissolving the food.

If testing points to problems with chewing, it usually means that the person needs to chew more thoroughly/slowly or leave time between mouthfuls.

If testing points to chewing each mouthful, it is not enough just to tell clients to 'chew more thoroughly'. You need to give them some guidance as to what this means. I usually ask the client how they want me to measure. You need to find a measurement that is meaningful to them. Possibilities include:

- Chew each mouthful for X seconds.
- Chew until the food is in a certain state.

So testing might look like this:

> *Do we need to look at Method Of Eating?* Yes
> *Do we need to look at chewing?* Yes
> *Is it the length of time Mary chews for?* Yes
> [Ask Mary how she'd like to measure this.]
> *So each mouthful should be chewed for at least five seconds?* Yes
> *At least 10 seconds?* No
> [Carry on asking questions to narrow it down.]

Time between mouthfuls is the other possibility. Some people just shovel food in at an amazing rate, barely finishing one mouthful before the next one goes in. So, the person may be chewing thoroughly enough, but not allowing any time to elapse between mouthfuls. There are several possibilities here:

- How long it would take them to eat a meal – you might want to test for several different meals so that they get some idea. E.g. your normal breakfast should take about 10 minutes, and your favourite meal (having asked them what that is) should take 25 minutes.
- Describe behaviour – putting the fork down between mouthfuls, not talking while they eat, counting to 10 between mouthfuls, etc.

This category often comes up for people who have digestive problems or need/want to lose weight. If food is eaten very quickly the full sensation does not get registered soon enough.

So a questioning session might look like this:

> *So we need to look at chewing?* Yes
> *Is it chewing each mouthful we are concerned with?* No
> *Is it time between mouthfuls?* Yes
> [Ask Sarah how she'd like to measure – how long to eat a meal or describing behaviour. In this case she goes for how long to eat a meal.]
> *So, how long to eat Sarah's typical breakfast – more than 10 minutes?* Yes
> *More than 15 minutes?* No
> [Etc.]

Sipping

This usually applies to liquids. It can refer to all liquids, just hot (or cold) ones, or to a particular liquid. Possibilities include sipping rather than gulping, or sipping more slowly. The easiest way to manage this is to establish through muscle testing what the client needs to do and then tell them to imagine doing it. You then ask if what they are imagining is correct. If it is not, you need to establish in what way it is incorrect, etc.

Smelling, Tasting And/Or Touching

Smelling Food: it may well be that making a conscious effort to smell food before eating can aid digestion.

Tasting Food: perhaps the client needs to taste a small portion of food and then wait before eating the rest.

Touching Food: This does not come up that often, but is always interesting when it does. I first thought about this sort of thing when I noticed that when I was very tired I tended to eat more with my fingers. I did some testing and came to the conclusion that lack of rest compromised my digestive system to some extent. Touching food in some way gave my body prior warning of what was coming, so that my stressed digestive system had more chance of doing the right thing with the food. As far as I know there is no known physiological mechanism by which touching food could affect the digestive juices, but it does not seem improbable. After all we evolved to eat with our hands and not with cutlery.

Whether you are looking at smelling, tasting or touching, the same sorts of questions are needed. Firstly it is important to see if this applies to all food. If not, check whether it is a particular type of food or meal or when people are experiencing generally high levels of stress or particular events. For example, in my case, it was something I had to do with all food whenever I was staying away from home for more than one night.

Eating With Conscious Awareness

Time between mouthfuls, smelling, tasting and touching the food can all be important ways of ensuring that the client eats with more conscious awareness of what they are doing, but sometimes this comes up in its own right. Many people eat while watching television, while reading a book or checking emails or while getting their children ready for school. The information may relate to a particular meal or to a particular activity, e.g.

Do we need information on eating with conscious awareness? Yes
Is it related to a particular meal? Yes
Is it breakfast? Yes
[Ask Pat how she eats her breakfast and she says she has a snack in the car while driving the children to school.).]
OK, does Pat need to be at home to eat her breakfast? Yes
Is it important whether this is before or after doing the school run? Yes
Is it before the school run? Yes
So does Pat need to sit down with the children and eat? Yes
Do we need to know more about this? Yes

Is it what Pat eats for breakfast? Yes
[Etc.]

Setting And Ritual

The setting in which we eat meals can be vitally important. Many people eat at tables covered with bills and things to do. A student on one course had a dying plant on the table that she had to remove as part of her nutritional homework.

Common things to come up here include:

- Eating in a particular place.

- Using particular cutlery or crockery.

- Using a tablecloth.

- Clearing the table of everything not to do with eating.

- Putting flowers on the table.

- Lighting a candle before eating.

- Saying affirmations before or after food.

- Making a blessing.

But, of course, there are many other possibilities that may also occur.

These requirements can relate to all meals or to one specific meal.

Body Position

I first became aware of this as a possibility because of personal experience. My eldest son was born with an exomphalos. This meant there was a large hole in his abdomen, and his large intestine had come through the hole and grown on the outside of his body. He had a major operation on the day he was born to put his intestines back inside his body and close the hole. When he was about eight he would not sit at the table to eat, but kept hopping off his chair and standing up to eat. We had a lot of arguments about this, but one day I started to wonder if he needed to stand up to eat. I did some muscle testing and found that he would benefit from standing to eat. Although the operation had been a success, it had not been possible to put his organs back into his body in exactly the correct place. While he was going through the current growth spurt this was causing him some discomfort and interfering with his proper digestion. Some time later when the growth spurt had ended, he began once again to sit to eat. This is, of course, an extreme example, but it may well be that other children and possibly adults would benefit from standing to eat.

A more common possibility is that people should not slouch while they are eating. The usual reason for this seems to be that it puts pressure inappropriately on our digestive organs. Sometimes they need to sit in a particular chair to eat, or just 'sit up properly'.

Temperature Of Food (02)

On the menu we have:

02 Temperature
- ➤ Too hot
  - ∗ All food and drink
  - ∗ All drink
  - ∗ All food
  - ∗ Category of food/drink
  - ∗ Particular food/drink
- ➤ Too cold
  - ∗ As above

Here we are not talking about the issue of raw or cooked, although eating only raw food will certainly mean that hot food is not eaten. The temperature requirement could mean either food must not be too cold or too hot or both. It can apply to food in general or a particular category of food or an individual food or drink. Testing will tell you which you need to look at in more detail.

Some people have a habit of eating beverages when they are just made even though they are really hot. Similarly some people eat food while it is very hot. The heat could affect the digestive system directly. It can also mean that people do not chew sufficiently as they transfer the hot food away from their mouth.

Clients may eat food too cold for their digestive system to work effectively. This can be a particular food (see page 17) or food in general.

Meals, Snacks And Timing (03 to 05)

On the menu we have:

03 Meals
- ➢ Number Of Meals
  - ＊ Increase
  - ＊ Decrease

04 Snacking
- ➢ Increase
- ➢ Decrease
- ➢ Specific foods

05 Timing
- ➢ Meals
  - ＊ All meals
  - ＊ One specific meal
- ➢ Earliest/latest time to eat
- ➢ Category of food
- ➢ One specific food
- ➢ Supplement(s)
- ➢ Drugs
- ➢ Other

Traditionally people have talked about three meals a day, but there is no evidence that this is the right number for everyone, although evidence does suggest that eating less than three meals a day leads to people eating high calorie and inappropriate foods when they do eat.

Increasing The Number Of Meals

This is most likely to occur if the client is having blood sugar problems (see page 200) or has problems combining foods (see page 103). This needs to be tested carefully to avoid the client gaining weight, unless, of course, this would be a positive outcome.

Decreasing The Number Of Meals

This does not occur very often, because usually people do not eat too many meals, but they may eat too many snacks.

Snacking

Some people are better if they eat throughout the day, whereas other people thrive better on regular meals at regular intervals. Testing will show whether the client should snack less or more. Sometimes it is important that the client snacks on a particular food at a particular time or related to a particular activity; e.g. eat an apple and drink half a litre of water one hour before going to the gym. Some people find they snack a lot because of cravings (see Appendix D).

Breakfast

There is evidence that missing breakfast is not a good idea. A lot of people miss breakfast because they are in a hurry or trying to lose weight. Eating breakfast often helps improve alertness and concentration through the morning and also reduces the chances of making inappropriate food choices later in the morning.

Eating Late In The Evening

Some clients benefit from this, as it helps to stabilise blood sugar through the night and allows them to wake more alert in the morning. If this comes up, it is usually important to determine what is eaten at this time. Some people do not benefit from eating late at night, as it leads to disturbed digestion and so disturbed sleep.

Using Affirmations To Control Eating

Affirmations can be extremely useful in lots of situations. If the client finds it difficult not to eat between meals even though this has been tested as the most appropriate thing to do, affirmations may help. Usually the affirmation is said out loud several times at the end of the meal. You need to test for the exact wording that would be appropriate for the client but examples would be:

- I've now finished eating till lunch/dinner/6.00 pm. (whatever is suitable given the circumstances)
- I have eaten enough food to last me till ...
- I'm full and do not need to eat till ...

Supplements And Timing

Various factors can affect the absorption of supplements, such as what is eaten or drunk at the same time, and the time of day. See Appendix A1 and A2 for more information.

Medication And Timing

Some drugs need to be taken with food, whereas others need to be taken on an empty stomach. In addition the interaction between drugs, foods and supplements is complex. Do bear in mind that it is illegal in many countries to advise people to ignore instructions given to them by the medical profession. If testing suggests that taking a particular drug with food (as prescribed by the doctor) is a problem, you need to deal with this in a sensitive way, probably suggesting that the person consults their doctor before making the tested changes. (For more on drugs and nutrition see Appendix D2.)

See page 40 for more information on timing.

Food Quality (06)

On the menu we have:

06 Food Quality
- ➤ Organic
- ➤ Freshness
- ➤ Other

Organic Food, Pesticides & Fungicides

Looking at the health risks of pesticides and fungicides is difficult, because many of the risks may be long term, and these can be difficult to establish. There are two basic problems: for the people who use them (the farm workers etc.) and for the people who may inadvertently consume them because they are present in food.

- **Organochlorides** kill pests by attacking their central nervous systems. Linked to cancer, birth defects and genetic changes in animals. They are fat-soluble and stored in body fat. They are far more persistent than organophosphates.

- **Organophosphates** interfere with nerve conduction in pests. They are the most common pesticide used today. They are water-soluble and break down rapidly.

- **Acaracides** are the class of pesticides used against mites and ticks.

The World Health Organisation, the European Union etc. have lists of banned and reduced-use chemicals. It is clear from research that some producers flout these standards and policing is very limited. The Pesticide Action Network UK (www.pan-uk.org) has more information on this.

As well as pesticides being harmful to humans in their own right, they may have other health implications. The use of synthetic fungicides prevents plants from producing salvestrols since they are not challenged by fungal infection. Salvestrols are anti-fungal compounds produced by the plant when fungal attack is likely. (Non-organic foods are usually low in salvestrols because they are sprayed with fungicides and so do not need to mount their own defence against attacks by fungus.) Salvestrols have been shown to be important anti-cancer compounds.

If organic food comes up as the category, you will need to check if this is for all food (or as close to that as the client can get practically) or for a specific food, food group, etc.

Freshness

Some people shop infrequently so that food can have lost a substantial amount of its nutrients and life force by the time it is consumed. Food that has been brought in from a long distance or left in the fridge for some time before consuming may be deficient in some nutrients. For example, water-soluble vitamins (B-group and C) are more unstable than fat-soluble vitamins (K, A, D and E) during food transporting and storage.

Sometimes there is a trade-off between freshness and organic. Local food may be fresher, but organic varieties may not be available. Testing will show which is more important for a particular client either in general or for a particular food.

Food Storage And Preparation (07)

On the menu we have:

07 Food Storage and Preparation
- ➤ Temperature of storage
  - * Fridge
  - * Freezer
  - * Particular food or category
- ➤ Light/Dark
- ➤ Containers, Wrappers And Utensils
  - * Phthalates
  - * Aluminium
  - * Nickel
  - * Lead
  - * Iron
  - * Clay
  - * Other
- ➤ Method of cooking
  - * Micro-waving
  - * Frying
  - * Other
- ➤ Other

Temperature Of Storage

Government guidelines for safe food storage are below 5 degrees centigrade in fridges and below minus 18 degrees centigrade in freezers. Many old fridges and freezers cannot maintain these temperatures easily, so testing may indicate the need for the purchase of a thermometer, so that temperatures can be checked and settings adjusted. Alternatively testing may indicate that a new appliance needs to be purchased.

Another possibility is that a particular food or food category should be stored in the fridge rather than in a cupboard or on display. This is particularly likely to apply to foods with a high oil content (e.g. nuts, seeds and cooking oils). Some people keep bottles of oil, herbs, etc. close to the cooker and this can be detrimental to the contents. It may be sufficient simply to move them further away from the cooker; testing will show what is necessary.

Light/Dark

Some foods should not be stored in the light from a nutritional point of view. This particularly applies to oils. As oils are usually better stored in the fridge, oil storage will often come up under the 'temperature of storage' category, and the need to store in the dark will automatically be met, but it may be that there are other foods that need to be stored in the dark (e.g. in a cupboard) for a particular client.

Containers, Wrappers And Utensils

Containers, wrappers and utensils do more than just hold the food. Molecules of substances can leach into the food. The ones that give cause for concern are:

- **Phthalates:** are used in the manufacturing of the softer plastics, particularly PVC, in printing inks and some adhesives. They can migrate from the packaging into the foodstuff. It is only recently that their ability to mimic oestrogen has been identified. This has been linked to falling sperm counts and breast cancer in humans. The UK Government insists that the levels in food are well within safety margins.

- **Aluminium:** common sources are aluminium cooking pans, aluminium foil and aluminium cans, particularly when the contents are drunk past their sell-by date. Also licensed as a food colouring, E173, but only for external decoration. Some anti-caking agents are aluminium based, (e.g. aluminium silicate), and these can be found in salt and baking powder, and as carry over ingredients in processed foods.

- **Nickel:** found in stainless steel cutlery etc. In theory, stainless steel is inert, but testing shows that some people who are allergic to nickel react to the nickel in stainless steel implements. The electrical elements in kettles also contain nickel. Hot drinks made from water boiled in a kettle where the element is in contact with the water will contain minute traces of nickel. May be in flour as a result of milling. Also used as a catalyst for hydrogenating vegetable oils.

- **Lead:** ceramic cookware may contain lead. Acidic foods such as oranges, tomatoes, or foods with vinegar will cause more lead to be leached from ceramic cookware than non-acidic foods like milk. More lead will leach into hot liquids like coffee, tea, and soups than into cold beverages. Any dishware that has a dusty or chalky grey residue on the glaze after it has been washed should not be used.

- **Iron:** cooking in an enamelled or uncoated cast iron pots increases the amount of iron in the diet, but this may not be in a form that is easily absorbed.

- **Clay:** crockery is usually made from clay, and by the time it is fired, it would seem unlikely that it would cause problems, but testing shows that some people who are allergic to clay react to crockery. People may also be sensitive to glazes.

Microwave Cooking

There appears to be no scientific evidence for the widely held view among CAM therapists that cooking or heating food in a microwave oven in some way "kills" it. This does not, of course, mean that there is no problem. It could be that the scientific evidence is not yet available. Objections to this form of cooking seem to be:

- It is an unnatural way to cook food: food is heated from the inside first, whereas in all traditional cooking methods food is heated from the outside first.

- Kirlian photography: Kirlian photographs show microwaved food with a different and less vibrant aura than conventionally cooked food.

- Many dowsers and kinesiologists say that microwaved foods tests differently.

If this came up in testing, you would need to test whether it applied to all food and drink, or to one or more specific foods or food categories.

Frying

Frying, particularly at high temperatures, can lead to the production of trans fatty acids (see page 83). Frying also increases production of free radicals (see page 98).

An Overview Of Metabolism

Metabolism involves:

- Catabolic processes - substances are broken down (e.g. turning proteins into amino acids).

- Anabolic processes - substances are built up (e.g. changing fatty acids and glycerol back into complex fats).

Both these processes are happening all the time as the body builds up new tissues and breaks down worn out ones. Anabolic processes require energy, which is provided by catabolic processes.

There are 7 essential categories of foods:

- Carbohydrate (see page 62)

- Protein (see page 71)

- Fats or lipids (see page 79)

- Water (see page 65)

- Vitamins (see page 90 and Appendix A1)

- Mineral salts (see page 94 and Appendix A2)

- Fibre (see page 69)

The vitamins and some of the minerals act to regulate tissue activity by playing a part in the enzyme system and so affect the health of the tissue. Water and mineral salts can be absorbed without digestion. Proteins, carbohydrates and fats have to be pre-digested in order to be used.

All the chemical and mechanical processes of digestion are aimed at changing the food into forms that can readily pass through the walls of the digestive tract and into the blood and lymph system. These forms are:

- Monosaccarides (starches and carbohydrate).

- Amino acids (protein).

- Fatty acids, glycerol and glycerides (oils and fats).

About 90% of absorption occurs in the small intestine. The rest is split between the stomach and the large intestine.

See appendix C for more detailed information on the digestive system.

Energy And Total Calories (08)

On the menu we have:

08 Total Calories
- ➤ Calories
  - ∗ Decrease
  - ∗ Increase
- ➤ Exercise (outside the scope of this book)

Calories And Energy Requirements

A calorie is a unit of heat energy. It is the amount of energy required to raise the temperature of 1 gm of water 1° C from $14.5 ^o$ C to $15.5 ^o$ C. The energy derived from food is measured in kilocalories (kcal). Kilocalories are also popularly known as calories. Kilojoules and mega joules are being used more and more as measures of energy.

1kcal = 4.2 kJ

Energy is needed for:

- The basic processes of life (e.g. breathing, metabolism, etc.)
- Muscular movement
- The creation of new tissues (growth and cell replacement)

Energy is derived from food. Protein, fat, carbohydrate and alcohol all contain chemical energy that can be transformed and used by the body. The body needs (has a physiological requirement for) carbohydrate, protein and fat, but no physiological requirement for alcohol.

- 1 gm of carbohydrate yields 4 kcal (17 kJ)
- 1 gm of protein yields 4 kcal (17 kJ)
- 1 gm of fat yields 9 kcal (37kJ)
- 1 gm of alcohol yields 7 kcal (29 kJ)

It takes about 3% of energy in the fat found in food to convert it to body fat.

It takes about 23% of energy in carbohydrate to convert it to body fat.

On average an adult man requires 2550 kcal per day and an adult woman 1940 kcal per day. This is a guideline only as there are enormous variations depending on activity levels, metabolic efficiency, etc. Energy needs increase for the repair necessary after surgery or severe injury.

Catabolism

The process of turning food into energy is called catabolism. The energy in the food needs to be released slowly in order for it to be used effectively. The end product of glucose metabolism is adenosine triphosphate (ATP), which is the form in which cells can utilise energy. There are three steps in this process, which take place within the cell in the mitochondrion:

- **Glycolysis** starts the process by converting glucose (or glycogen) into pyruvate and produces a small amount of ATP, without the need for oxygen. If oxygen is present then acetyl CoA is produced which enters the Krebs cycle.

- **Krebs cycle** (also called citric acid cycle or tricarboxylic acid cycle) uses oxygen and converts acetyl CoA into carbon dioxide, water and hydrogen.

- **Electron transfer pathway** uses oxygen and releases the energy in the hydrogen to produce ATP and heat with the by-product of water.

If the energy supply from food is less than the body needs then it will use its own tissues to provide energy. Initially this will come from body fat, but eventually muscles will be used as an energy source. The muscles used will include those from vital organs such as the heart. Eventually there will be organ dysfunction leading to death.

If the energy supply from food is more than it needs then the surplus will be stored as fat.

Decreasing And Increasing Total Calories

This particular item does not come up very often. I suspect that this is because it is rarely a matter of just altering or reducing calories. Clients might follow the instruction 'reduce calories' by reducing nutritious foods and keeping in foods that offer little nutrition. Similarly if someone has to increase calories it is likely to be important that they do not just add chocolate, alcohol and sugar. If this category does come up, bear in mind the issues around replacements and additions (see page 19).

Often the result of nutritional testing means that calories are reduced indirectly through some intervention elsewhere in the nutritional menu. For example, if testing shows that the amount of raw food in the diet needs to be increased, this may lead to a natural reduction in calorie consumption, even though that has not been explicitly stated. Many clients respond better to an instruction to increase something (even if it is 'only' raw food) than decrease something (total calories). Testing seems to take into account this predisposition of clients.

All the evidence is that people who focus on reducing calories may be successful in the short run at losing weight, but in the long run the 'diet mentality' breaks down and people return to their old habits, so this may be why this category comes up so rarely.

One possibility for people who find it difficult to put on weight is that total calorie consumption is manipulated by decreasing calories for a while and then increasing calories. You would need to test for the exact number of days/weeks for each phase. This is, of course, the classic behaviour of yo-yo dieting that does not help people to lose weight, but tends to lead to weight gain in the long run. Here, through appropriate testing, it is usefully being applied for people who want to gain weight.

Carbohydrate And The Glycaemic Index (09)

On the menu we have:

09 Carbohydrate And The Glycaemic Index
- ➢ Increase carbohydrate generally
- ➢ Decrease carbohydrate generally
- ➢ Increase low glycaemic index foods
  - ✱ Specific food(s)
  - ✱ In general
  - ✱ Time of day
  - ✱ Activity related
- ➢ Decrease low glycaemic index foods
  - ✱ As above
- ➢ Increase high glycaemic index foods
  - ✱ As above
- ➢ Decrease high glycaemic index foods
  - ✱ As above

If the carbohydrates (starch) in food were burnt directly, there would be too sudden a release of energy as heat, and not enough energy for body processes.

Most of the carbohydrates we eat are polysaccharides (such as potatoes and cereals) or disaccharides (such as are found in fruit, sugar, honey and milk). Neither of these can be absorbed into the blood stream, as the molecules are too large, but monosaccharides are small enough to be absorbed. So, polysaccharides and disaccharides have to be changed into monosaccharides such as glucose, galactose and fructose in order to be absorbed.

Polysaccharides are complex carbohydrates, whereas disaccharides and monosaccharides are simple carbohydrates.

In the mouth salivary amylase (also called ptyalin) breaks the chemical bonds to create maltose. Usually the food is swallowed too quickly for this process to be completed, but some of the amylase is swallowed with the food and continues acting on it in the stomach until the stomach acids inactivate it.

Pancreatic amylase in the small intestine continues the process of digesting carbohydrates. Maltase, sucrase and lactase change maltose, sucrose and lactose into simpler sugars (glucose, fructose, galactose and lactose), which can then be absorbed. Any remaining carbohydrate is digested by fermentation in the large intestine.

Fructose and galactose are converted into glucose by the liver. Glucose not needed for immediate use may be converted to glycogen by the liver. Glucose is soluble in water and so is readily transported around the body through the bloodstream.

Glycogen is insoluble in water. It is stored in the liver itself and in skeletal muscle fibres. If there is not enough room to store all the glycogen it is converted into fat and stored in adipose tissues. The body can store fats more efficiently than it can store glucose.

When the body needs these stores for energy, the glycogen and fat are transformed back into glucose. The cells of the body use the glucose to provide energy. The hormone insulin secreted by the pancreas allows the cells to burn glucose for energy and the liver to store excess glucose as glycogen. (See appendix D3.)

The Glycaemic Index

It used to be thought that complex carbohydrates (starches) were absorbed more slowly than simple carbohydrates (sugars). This was based on the assumption that complex carbohydrates would be harder to digest, as they were larger molecules. Work by Professor David Jenkins showed that some starch foods give an equivalent blood-sugar response to some simple sugars.

From this work he developed the glycaemic index. This index is a measure of food's effect on blood sugar. Glucose has a G. I. Value of 100. Foods with a high glycaemic index will tend to lead to a rapid surge in blood sugar levels and mean that the pancreas has to work harder:

Apple Juice: 40
Apple: 38
Apricots, dried: 31
Apricots, fresh: 64
Banana: 55
Biscuits: 62-79
Bread, rye (pumpernickel): 41
Bread, white: 70
Bread, wholemeal: 69
Breakfast cereals, sweetened: 77- 84
Broad beans: 79
Buckwheat: 54
Bulgar: 48
Cakes: 44-76
Carrots: 49
Cherries: 22
Chick peas: 33
Chocolate: 49-68

Croissant: 67
Grapes: 46
Honey: 58
Kiwi Fruit: 52
Lentils: 28
Low fat yoghurt: 33
Lucozade: 95
Milk: 27-32
Orange juice: 46
Orange squash: 66
Orange: 44
Parsnips: 97
Pasta: 32-41
Pastry, flaky: 59
Peaches: 42
Peanuts: 14
Peas: 48
Pineapple: 66

Pitta Bread: 57
Porridge: 42 (not one-minute variety)
Potato crisps: 54
Potato: 56-83
Raisins: 64
Rice Cakes: 82
Rice, Basmati: 58
Rice, brown: 76

Rice, white: 87
Ryvita Rye Crispbread: 69
Sausages: 28
Sports Drinks: 70-80
Sucrose: 65
Sultanas: 56
Sweet corn: 55
Yoghurt, low-fat fruit: 33

Each food has to be tested separately: similar foods can have dramatically different GI indexes. This is partly dependent on how easy it is for the enzymes to break down the starch, e.g. one type of starch, amylopectin, has more branches to its structure and so is easier to digest than amylose, another type. The physical structure can also have an effect. For example, the exploded structure of bread and rice cakes gives more surfaces for the enzymes to work on than does pasta. Also the body can break down sucrose more easily than it can fructose (fruit sugar).

In general a meal made up of several different foods will have a GI index based on the proportion of each food and its GI index, so it is possible to predict the GI index of a meal if the information for the individual components is known.

The GI index can produce some anomalies. For example, suggesting that it is better to eat a chocolate bar than a slice of wholemeal bread. The GI index of a food is only one aspect of its nutritional role. People sometimes look at this chart and say something like: "So, cake is better for me than parsnips." But other factors are also important, e.g. fibre content (see page 69), vitamin and mineral content, etc., so this chart should not be used alone in considering what constitutes a healthy diet.

Low GI foods contribute to endurance and help to control mood swings (see page 199) and variations in energy levels. High glycaemic index foods aid recovery after exercise.

Water (10)

On the menu we have:

10 Water
- ➤ Quantity
  - * In relation to meals
  - * In relation to a food category
  - * In relation to a specific food
  - * In relation to an activity
  - * Other
- ➤ Quality
- ➤ Timing (see page 40)
- ➤ Other

Functions Of Water

The body is about 60% water by weight. Water acts as:

- A solvent which assists in the break down and transport of other substances

- A coolant and so helps to maintain a constant body temperature

- A lubricating fluid – it is a component of mucus, synovial fluid in joint cavities, saliva etc.

Water Quantity

Water is more vital than food: it is only possible to live for a few days without water. Most of the body's water needs are met from liquids but some does come from solids. Some food contains a large amount of water, e.g. apples are over 80% water, eggs and potatoes over 70%, and even sultanas are almost 20% water. Even so, I have never had increasing water quantity by increasing the quantity of water-rich foods come up in testing.

Many people rely on tea, coffee and alcohol for their water intake. Tea and coffee act as a diuretic. It has been suggested by some practitioners that more water is excreted from the body than is taken in when a cup of coffee or tea is drunk, but there appears to be no scientific evidence for this. See Dr F Batmanghelidj's book *Your Body's Many Cries For Water* for a more detailed discussion of the importance of water.

A rough guide for most people is to check the colour of the urine – pale straw-coloured urine indicates an adequate intake of water, although B vitamin supplements and some drugs will colour the urine. Testing can provide more detailed information, e.g.

Are we looking at water? Yes
Water quantity? Yes

Water Quality, Taps/Faucets

Water quality from taps/faucets can be affected by:

- Hormones from the contraceptive pill, and organic solvents from industrial processes.

- Pesticides and fertilizers, as run-off from farmland.

- Heavy metals, such as aluminium, zinc and lead, are only really a problem in soft water areas because there they can dissolve into the water.

- Aluminium sulphate is sometimes added to the water supply to remove particles from the water. Normally most of the aluminium sulphate will be removed as it combines with the particles and falls out of the water as sediment. The levels of aluminium remaining are very low, but will affect some people.

- Trihalomethanes can also be present in the water - formed in small amounts when chlorine and natural organic matter in the water interact. Chloroform is a trihalomethane, these substances have been associated with cancers and allergies.

- In some areas peat will be suspended in the water. This is probably not a general health hazard, but it can affect taste and colour of the water.

- Water pipes used to be made from galvanised zinc – iron coated with zinc; these pipes can break down over many years, releasing zinc into the water supply.

- In some areas rust will be coming off the pipes.

- Some old pipes in the UK that run under farmland are made from asbestos. Sometimes farm machinery will damage a part of the pipe, so the water board will cut that piece out and replace it with a piece of new plastic pipe but leave the rest of the old asbestos pipe in place.

Modern pipes are mainly made from polythene, and concern has been expressed about phthalates (see page 55) leaching from the plastic. Some people also show an allergic reaction to this. (Much of the information above from Ken Digby of NT Laboratories Ltd.)

It is not necessary to test why the individual needs to be using a water filter or bottled water rather than tap water, but this information is useful background information.

Water Quality, Bottled Water

The National Resources Defense Council had over 1000 bottles of water independently tested and say on their web site: "Our conclusion is that there is no assurance that just because water comes out of a bottle it is any cleaner or safer than water from the tap. And in fact, an estimated 25 percent or more of bottled water is really just tap water in a bottle - sometimes further treated, sometimes not." (www.nrdc.org)

The plastic bottles may be made from PET (polyethylene terephthalate). Antimony trioxide is used in the manufacture of this plastic and small amounts of antimony can migrate into the water before it is drunk.

Water Quality, Filters

Water authorities have to operate to certain legal standards, and they will often say that the levels of certain chemicals are below the limits set by WHO, but nevertheless a lot of people feel healthier if they use filtered water.

There are various filters on the market. Some are jug systems and some are plumbed in. Most filters use carbon to remove hormones, pesticides and solvents.

Types of filter:

- **Granular activated carbon**: contains a resin which is good at removing calcium carbonate – this is found in hard water areas and gives the 'scum' on top of your cup of tea.

- **Carbon block**: is more efficient than the granulated filter because the particles are very small so there is more surface area for the water to come into contact with. You can use this system to filter all the water in your house, not just the drinking water. They will remove hormones, pesticides, organic solvents and nitrates. Some are impregnated with other materials and so will also remove heavy metals.

- **Carbon block filter plus silver**: prevents the growth of bacteria and algae. Particularly good when the filter is only going to be used intermittently with many days or weeks in between uses.

- **Reverse osmosis**: Forces water through a very fine membrane under pressure. It removes everything dissolved in the water, so you get very pure water. In general you need a carbon filter as well, otherwise too much organic material will get through and contaminate the RO membrane. This will be a breeding ground for bacteria. This is also why RO systems need to left running all the time. If you stop the process, the membrane becomes contaminated. In general you need to change the membrane once a year. These filters also remove nutritional salts – such as calcium and magnesium salts - that are dissolved in the water. These are left in by carbon filters.

Testing For Water Quality

People do not usually drink the same water all the time, e.g. home/work; tap/filtered/bottled, so you need to establish first what water you're talking about before you start testing a client. For example:

Are we looking at water? Yes
Water quantity? No
Water quality? Yes
[Check with the client to see if he uses the same water supply all the time. The client says that he uses a jug filter at home, tap water at work and bottled water when out and about.]
So do we need to look at the water drunk at home? No
The water drunk at work? Yes
[Etc.]

The quality of a client's water intake may be improved by:

- Using a water filter.

- Changing to a different type of filter.

- Changing the filter of their existing system more often.

- Using bottled water.

- Using tap water.

So to carry on with the previous example:

What would be best – to bring filtered water in from home? No
To use bottled water? Yes
Is there a preference for the brand of water? Yes
Is this one or more of the brands that John drinks now when he's out and about? Yes
[Etc.]

Fibre (11)

On the menu we have:

11 Fibre
- ➢ Soluble
  - * Increase
  - * {Decrease} - **unlikely**
- ➢ Insoluble
  - * Increase
  - * Decrease

Fibre Intake

At one time fibre was thought to serve no useful purpose in the body, as it does not contain any nutrients, but it is now recognised that fibre performs important functions. Total fibre intake should be around 18g a day on average, but many people get less than 12g a day (British Nutrition Foundation). There are two types of fibre: insoluble and soluble:

- Insoluble Fibre: found in wholemeal bread, wholemeal pasta, brown rice, vegetables - especially beans, peas and lentils - nuts and dried fruit. It binds with water in various ways, but does not dissolve in water.

- Soluble Fibre: found in oats, barley, rye, pulses and fruit. It can dissolve in water.

Fibre Content Of Food

The main constituent of fibre is non-starch polysaccharides. Fibre is only available from foods of plant origin. Examples of fibre content:

Wheat bran 48 g of fibre per 100 g (3.5 oz)
Whole-wheat 11 g of fibre per 100 g
Cooked carrots 3.7 g of fibre per 100 g
Raw frozen peas 7.75 g of fibre per 100 g
1 medium apple provides about 1.8g
100g (3.5 oz) brown rice provides about 0.8g
100g (3.5 oz) baked beans provides 3.5g
1 bowl of porridge provides about 1.8g

Benefits Of Fibre

There are many benefits of eating a diet high in fibre:

- Fibre bulks up stools and so reduces constipation.

- Fibre keeps the intestinal wall clean and reduces the likelihood of developing diverticulitis.

- Bacteria in the colon can break down fibre, creating an acidic environment that decreases the risk of developing colorectal cancer.

- A high fibre intake can increase the beneficial bacteria population. (See page 101)

- Foods high in fibre can take longer to eat, increasing the feeling of fullness after a meal, and so help weight control.

- Food high in fibre is digested more slowly and so glucose may be released more slowly into the blood stream.

- Soluble fibre binds with cholesterol, so lowering blood cholesterol levels. (See page 87)

Disadvantages Of Fibre

There are some disadvantages of fibre.

- Fibre can bind with some minerals such as iron and reduce their absorption. Phytic acid is found in the hulls of nuts, seeds, and grains. It binds with calcium, magnesium, iron, and zinc and stops them being absorbed.

- Clients who are already suffering from inflammatory gut problems (e.g. diverticulitis, Crohn's disease, etc.) may not benefit from an increase in fibre, as this can physically aggravate the existing inflammation.

Protein (12)

On the menu we have:

12 Protein
- ➢ Overall quantity
  - * Increase
  - * Reduce
- ➢ Particular type of protein
  - * Increase
  - * Reduce
- ➢ Particular amino acid
  - * Increase
  - * Reduce
- ➢ Timing (see page 40)

Proteins

Proteins are made up of simpler substances called amino acids (see page 73). The protein in food is first broken down in the stomach by the enzyme pepsin. Then, in the small intestine, trypsin, chymotrypsin, carboxypeptidase in the pancreatic juices carry on the work, converting them into amino acids. The amino acids pass through the gut wall and can then be re-built into the proteins that the body needs.

Although cells synthesise many different chemicals, a large part of the cellular machinery is devoted to producing proteins. Proteins determine the physical and chemical characteristics of cells and so are vitally important. Proteins are used to produce:

- Enzymes
- Some hormones
- Organelles (cellular machinery)
- Muscle (e.g. actin and myosin)
- Structural components of skin and hair (e.g. collagen and keratin)
- Plasma (blood) protein
- Antibodies

The instructions for producing proteins are coded within the genes.

It is possible for the body also to use proteins for energy, but it is not its first choice. Protein is essential for the body, as it is the only type of food that contains nitrogen. Excess protein is converted into fat or glycogen or glucose.

Food Protein Content

No food is just protein, although some foods have a higher proportion of protein than others. The actual protein content varies depending on growing and rearing conditions, climate etc, so these figures are a guide only:

- Meat 20-30 % protein
- Whole grains 10% protein
- Cheese 25% protein
- Cows milk 3% protein
- Nuts 15-25% protein
- Pulses about 7%

In practical terms this means:

- 85 grams (3 ounces) of meat has around 23 grams of protein
- 113g (4 ounces) of tofu has approximately 8g of protein
- A quarter litre of milk has approximately 8g of protein
- 39g (1.3 ounces) of peanuts provides 10g of protein
- 385g (13.5 ounces) boiled brown rice provides about 10g of protein

Dietary Requirements For Protein

There are large amounts of variation in the amount of protein people eat. It is difficult to establish the minimum amount of protein people need because there are no definitive deficiency signs apart from growth failure and tissue wasting, which are extreme signs. The UK Reference Nutrient Intake (the amount of nutrient which is thought to be enough for at least 97% of the population) for protein per day is now:

- 53 to 55 g per day for men
- 45 - 46.5 g for women
- 51g for pregnant women

- 53 to 56g for breast feeding women
- 28.3 g for children aged 7-10 years

The recommended amounts of protein for adults and children has more than halved in the last 20 years. So the current figure should not be taken as absolutely right.

People who get all their protein from plant sources may need to increase this slightly (multiplying by 1.1 is the standard advice), as plant proteins can be less digestible.

Regular exercisers do not usually need to increase their protein intake: "There is no evidence that habitual exercise increases protein requirements; indeed protein metabolism may become more efficient as a result of training." (Annual Review Of Nutrition, 2000;20:457-83.)

High Protein Weight Loss Diets

High protein diets have been seen as a good way of losing weight, but research suggests that the benefits may be temporary. Initially weight loss tends to be great as water is lost from the body with the reduction in carbohydrate. In theory a high protein diet could put a strain on the kidneys. High protein diets have also been linked to bone-density loss. (See acid and alkaline balance, page 107.)

For people wishing to lose weight eating small amounts of protein throughout the day may be beneficial as this stimulates metabolism, and gives a sense of fullness. It is important to make sure that fat intake is not increased along with any additional increase in protein.

Long-term results from the European Prospective Investigation into Cancer and Nutrition (EPIC) show that high-protein, low-carbohydrate diets increase mortality risk. Researchers assessed the diets of 22,944 healthy Greek adults. Those consuming diets highest in protein and lowest in carbohydrate had a 22 percent greater risk of death, compared with those consuming diets highest in carbohydrate and lowest in protein. (Trichopoulou A, Psaltopoulou T, Orfanos P, Hsieh C-C, Trichopoulos D. Low-carbohydrate-high-protein diet and long-term survival in a general population cohort. *European Journal of Clinical Nutrition* 2007;61:575-581.)

Amino Acids

Proteins are made from amino acids. In the body, proteins (in food) are broken down into amino acids and then reassembled to form other proteins suitable for the human body. There are approximately 250,000 different human proteins.

Amino acids are stored in the liver until needed and then synthesised in the relevant cells and tissues into the correct proteins. The amino acids can be re-built into the proteins that the body needs.

Amino acids are divided into:

- Essential (cannot be manufactured by the body and, therefore, must be taken in food)

- Non-essential – this does not mean that they are unnecessary. It means that the body can manufacture them, so it is not essential to get them from food.

Large amounts of essential amino acids are found in meat and dairy foods. Non-animal sources of protein vary in which essential amino acids they contain. E.g. cereals lack lysine, and pulses lack methionine, but, by combining different ones (e.g. cereals and nuts/pulses) a meal can contain all the essential amino acids. So, in practice a variety of protein sources will provide all the essential amino acids. It was thought at one time that the different amino acids needed to be eaten at the same time in order to make a complete protein, but this is now recognised to be incorrect.

D and L Forms Of Amino Acids

Amino acids can be in two forms: D & L. This is often likened to humans being right handed or left handed. Biological processes occurring in the body involve molecules recognising each other in some way. In general the human body does not recognise and therefore cannot use the D form of amino acids, although the body can utilise D-phenylalanine. For this reason any amino acid supplements should be of the L form., and you will see them listed as L-glutathione, etc.

Functions Of Amino Acids And Good Sources

Animal proteins include all amino acids so are not listed, but there are also many excellent non-animal sources of protein.

	Functions And Correlations	Good Non-Animal Sources Include	
Alanine	Involved in the metabolism of tryptophan and the vitamin B6.	Beans, nuts, seeds, soya, brewer's yeast, brown rice bran, corn, legumes, whole grains.	

	Functions And Correlations	Good Non-Animal Sources Include	
Arginine	Stimulates human growth hormone which stimulates defence function; accelerates wound healing; detoxifying ammonia; normal sperm count; glucose control mechanism in blood; enhances fat metabolism; involved in insulin production; arthritis; inhibition of tumour development; premature ageing; overweight; fatigue; memory.	Peanuts, tofu, pumpkin seed, almonds, sunflower seeds, Brazil nuts, chocolate, cereals	Essential for children but not for adults.
Asparagine	Required by the nervous system and in the synthesis of ammonia.	Asparagus, potatoes, legumes, nuts, seeds, soya, whole grains	Non-essential
Aspartic Acid	Protects liver; detoxification of ammonia; promotes uptake of trace elements in the gut; involved in the energy cycle; involved in transportation of magnesium and potassium.		Non-essential
Cystine/ Cysteine	Part of insulin molecule; heavy metal chelator; psoriasis; eczema; tissue healing after surgery.	Soya protein, almonds, sesame seeds, walnuts.	Essential for children but not for adults.
Glutamic Acid/Glutamate	Precursor of proline, ornithine, arginine and polyamines; a stimulatory neurotransmitter; can be converted in body into GABA (inhibitory neurotransmitter); nearly all excitatory neurons in the CNS and possibly half of the synapses in the brain communicate via glutamate; visual adaptation to light and dark; many epileptics have increased levels of glutamic acid; part of the acute reaction to withdrawal from drug addiction includes increase production of glutamate.		Non-essential
Glutamine	Dominant amino acids in cerebro-spinal fluid and serum; passes through blood/brain barrier; powerful "brain fuel"; gives rise to GABA which is a calming agent; helps maintain body's nitrogen level; used in production of other non-essential amino acids; protects from alcohol; reduces desire for alcohol and sometimes sugar; heals peptic ulcers; depression; blunts carbohydrate craving; hypoglycaemia; schizophrenia; senility; fatigue; memory improvement; concentration; smoking.		Non-essential

	Functions And Correlations	Good Non-Animal Sources Include	
Glycine	Can be synthesised from other amino acids (serine and threonine); acts as an inhibitory neurotransmitter; assists in manufacture of DNA, glycerol, phospholipids, collagen, glutathione and cholesterol conjugates; essential for one of key liver detoxification pathways; stimulates secretion of glucagons; in spinal cord (inhibitory action) and in retina; Parkinson's disease; low levels often found in manic-depressives and epileptics. People with motor neurone disease may have impaired glycine metabolism and have high levels of glycine in the blood.		Non-essential
Histidine	Metabolised into histamine which is important for smooth muscle function and contraction and expansion of blood vessels; sexual arousal; auditory nerve function; stimulates production of red and white blood cells; schizophrenia; protects against radiation damage; chelates toxic metals; rheumatoid arthritis; digestive tract ulcers; nausea during pregnancy; hearing problems; allergies; anxiety; low stomach acid; smoking.	Soya protein concentrate, peanuts, tofu, sunflower seeds.	Essential for children but not for adults
Isoleucine	Chronically sick; formation of haemoglobin; energy production; reduces tremors and twitching in animals; body building.	Soya protein concentrates, soya flour, tofu, peanuts, almonds, pumpkin seeds, sunflower seeds.	Essential
Leucine	Chronically sick; essential for growth; wound healing of skin and bones; energy production; Parkinson's disease; enhances effects of endorphins.	Soya protein concentrate, soya flour, peanuts, tofu, almonds, pumpkin seeds.	Essential
Lysine	Often low in vegetarian diets; important for children's growth and development; involved in synthesis of carnitine, so important in fat metabolism; formation of antibodies; dietary deficiency leads to increased calcium excretion; herpes simplex; concentration; fatigue; dizziness; anaemia; visual disorders; nausea; hypoglycaemia.	Soya protein concentrate, soya flour, tofu, parsley, quinoa, whole-wheat flour.	Essential

	Functions And Correlations	Good Non-Animal Sources Include	
Methionine	Antioxidant preventing free radical damage; helps produce choline, adrenaline, lecithin and B12; assists gallbladder function; precursor of taurine, cystine and cysteine. Heavy metal and histamine detoxifier; strengthens hair follicles; detoxifies liver; affects selenium bio-availability; arthritic and rheumatoid symptoms; detoxification; antioxidation; retards cataracts; Parkinson's disease; schizophrenia; gallbladder problems resulting from use of contraceptive oestrogen; poor skin tone; hair loss; anaemia; retarded protein synthesis; atherosclerosis; herpes; memory; premature ejaculation.	Brazil nuts, sunflower seeds, sesame seeds, beans, lentils, soya beans, quinoa.	Essential
Phenylalanine	Precursor of tyrosine and therefore dopamine, norepinephrine (noradrenaline) and epinephrine (adrenaline), so affects heart rate, blood pressure, oxygen consumption, blood sugar levels, fat metabolism; important for brain; necessary for thyroid; shortage predisposes children to eczema; weight control; antidepressant; pain killer; MS; Parkinson's disease; memory; concentration and mental alertness; rheumatoid arthritis; vitiligo; emotional disorders; circulatory problems; drug addiction; tremors.	Soya protein concentrate, soya flour, tofu, peanuts, almonds, sesame seeds, sunflower seeds.	Essential
Proline	Production of collagen and cartilage.		Non-essential
Serine	Can be made in human body from glycine; used to make substances such as choline, phospholids, phosphotidylserine; present in all cell membranes; plays a key role in membrane stability.	Gluten, soya, peanuts.	Non-essential
Threonine	Necessary for formation of teeth enamel protein, elastin and collagen; minor role controlling fat build up in liver; precursor of glycine and serine; immune stimulating as promotes thymus growth and activity; digestive and intestinal tract functioning; indigestion; malabsorption; irritability; personality disorders.	Soya protein concentrate, soya flour, tofu, peanuts, almonds.	Essential

	Functions And Correlations	Good Non-Animal Sources Include	
Tryptophan	Synthesis of B3; precursor of serotonin; mood stabiliser; vascular migraine, anti-depressant; weight control; sleep enhancer; menopausal depression; pain killer; restless leg syndrome; rheumatoid arthritis; tardive dyskinesia; mental disturbances, depression, brittle finger nails; poor skin colouring and tone; indigestion; carbohydrate craving. May aggravate bronchial asthma and lupus.	Soya protein concentrate, soya flour, tofu, almonds, peanuts, pumpkin seeds, sesame seeds, tahini, almonds, sunflower seeds.	Essential
Tyrosine	Derived from phenylalanine; precursor of thyroid hormones, dopa, dopamine, norepinephrine and epinephrine; aids normal brain function; Parkinson's disease; depression; increasing brain neurotransmitter levels; alleviating hay fever and grass allergies; drug addiction; tremors; low blood pressure.	Soya protein concentrate, soya flour, tofu, almonds, pumpkin seeds, peanuts, peanut butter.	Essential for children but not for adults.
Valine	Helpful in treating addictions; deficiency may affect myelin covering of nerves; energy; muscle building and c-ordination; liver and gallbladder disease; mental function; nervousness; poor sleep patterns; excess gives skin crawling sensations and hallucinations.	Soya protein concentrate, soya flour, tofu, pumpkin seeds, peanuts.	Essential

Oils And Fats (13)

On the menu we have:

13 Oils And Fats
- ➢ Saturated fats
  - ∗ Increase in general
  - ∗ Increase specific one(s)
  - ∗ Decrease in general
  - ∗ Decrease specific one(s)
- ➢ Polyunsaturated fats
  - ∗ Increase in general
  - ∗ Increase specific one(s)
  - ∗ Decrease in general
  - ∗ Decrease specific one(s)
- ➢ Monounsaturated fats
  - ∗ Increase in general
  - ∗ Increase specific one(s)
  - ∗ Decrease in general
  - ∗ Decrease specific one(s)
- ➢ Transfatty acids
  - ∗ {Increase in general} - **unlikely**
  - ∗ {Increase specific one(s)} - **unlikely**
  - ∗ Decrease in general
  - ∗ Decrease specific one(s)
- ➢ Omega-3 Fatty Acids
  - ∗ Increase in food
  - ∗ Increase as a supplement
  - ∗ Decrease in food
  - ∗ Decrease as a supplement
- ➢ Omega-6 Fatty Acids
  - ∗ Increase in food
  - ∗ Increase as a supplement
  - ∗ Decrease in food
  - ∗ Decrease as a supplement
- ➢ Omega-9 Fatty Acids
  - ∗ Increase in food
  - ∗ Increase as a supplement
  - ∗ Decrease in food
  - ∗ Decrease as a supplement
- ➢ Custom Oil Blend

Fats

The main digestion of fats occurs in the small intestine where pancreatic lipase is active. Bile helps to emulsify fats. Fats from food are broken down into their parts (fatty acids and monoglycerides) and then reassembled in intestinal cells. They then pass into the lymphatic system and eventually flow into the bloodstream. After another round of breakdown and reassembly (with the help of insulin), the fat molecules make it into fat cells.

In the stomach gastric lipase breaks down the butterfat in milk to produce fatty acids and monoglycerides. This enzyme needs a level of stomach acidity that is found in small children but not in adults.

Functions of Fats

The main uses of fats in the body are:

- To make membranes including cell membranes.

- To act as signalling molecules (messenger molecules).

- To transport other molecules, e.g. vitamin A

- As a back-up source of energy. The body prefers to use carbohydrates (see page 62) because these are easier to break down than fats, but as fat is energy dense large amounts of energy can be stored as fat.

If there is no immediate use for the fats, they are stored in the liver and in the adipose tissues as fat.

Although some popular diets suggest that fat is always a problem because of its high calorific value, adequate lipid consumption is necessary for health. Fats are used in the building of some tissues, e.g. nerve tissue and marrow. Lipids consist of essential fatty acids that cannot be synthesised in the body.

Essential Fatty Acids

Fatty acids are classified as essential or non-essential depending on whether the body is able to synthesise them. Essential fatty acids are important because the body uses them to make hormone-like substances called prostaglandins that are vital for good health. They are also used to make nerve cells and cellular membranes.

There are two groups of essential fatty acids distinguished by their structures: omega-6 and omega-3. The main sources of these are in polyunsaturated vegetable oils and fish oils. Some supplements also contain these.

Omega-3 Fatty Acids

The major source is fish. The main vegetarian sources of omega-3 fatty acids are linseed oil (also known as flax seed oil) and pumpkin seeds. Small amounts are also found in walnuts, wheat germ and soya oil. In recent years high levels of mercury have been found in fish, so the use of fish oil supplements has been brought into question.

The fish oils are already in the form of eicosapentaenoic acid (EPA) and docosahexaenoic acid (DHA). The vegetarian sources produce alpha-linolenic acid (ALA), which is converted into EPA. There is also some evidence that some must be converted into DHA as well. EPA and DHA affect blood clotting and may help to prevent thrombosis.

EPA appears also to reduce the inflammatory response of the body and so can be helpful in conditions such as rheumatoid arthritis. Omega-3 deficiencies can lead to behavioural problems, muscle weakness, visual impairment, rheumatic and arthritic problems.

Omega-6 Fatty Acids

Sunflower and sesame oils are good sources of omega-6 fatty acids. The main omega-6 fatty acid is linoleic acid. Gamma-linolenic acid (GLA) and arachidonic acid are derived from it. These affect inflammatory processes, the immune system and hormone balance.

Omega-6 deficiency can lead to eczema, psoriasis, hair loss, infertility, weight gain, behavioural and circulatory problems. Smoking, alcohol, viral infections, eating a lot of saturated fats, being short of zinc, magnesium and vitamin B_6 may reduce enzyme activity along this pathway.

Some people have problems with the conversion process within the body. Signs of this can include hyperactivity, thirst and small bumps on the upper arm. Supplements of evening primrose oil and starflower oil (borage oil) supply GLA and so by-pass one of the steps in the conversion. These can be useful for people who have problems with the conversion process.

Some recent research has focussed on conjugated linoleic acid (CLA), a fatty acid found mainly in milk fat and meat. CLA is in short supply in the modern diet, because of changes to the way cattle are reared and the move to skimmed milk. Experiments feeding human and animals CLA supplements have shown an increase in body muscle and a decrease in body fat. CLA has also been shown to inhibit tumour formation and suppress atherosclerosis in experimental animals. CLA is available as a supplement.

Omega-9 Fatty Acids

These are not considered essential, as the body can make them. Fats in this family include oleic acid, erucic acid and stearic acid. Oleic acid is the main component of olive oil and is also found in avocadoes and nuts such as almond and cashew. Erucic acid is found in rapeseed and mustard seed. Stearic acid is prevalent in large quantities in animal fats.

Types of Dietary Fat

There are three types of dietary fats:

- Saturated fats (SFA's).

- Polyunsaturated fats (PUFAs).

- Monounsaturated fats (MFAs).

Most authorities agree that the typical Western diet contains too much fat in total and that the balance between the different fatty acids is not correct. Contrary to what much of the media say, not <u>all</u> fats are bad.

All dietary fats contain a mixture of the three types of fatty acids: saturated, polyunsaturated and monounsaturated, but the proportions vary, so that sources are classified by their predominant fat.

In unsaturated fats not all the chemical bonds are linked to hydrogen atoms. This allows the formation of double bonds within the fat molecule, giving these oils a much more flexible structure.

Saturated Fats (SFAs)

These occur mainly in animal foods and are hard at room temperature. They can be synthesised by the body These include meat, dairy products, coconut and palm oil. These are converted into LDL-cholesterol (see page 87). Saturated fats increase the stickiness of the blood making thrombosis more likely and interfere with the function of essential fatty acids (see page 80).

Polyunsaturated Fats (PUFAs)

These include corn oil, evening primrose oil, grape seed oil, safflower oil, sesame oil, soya oil, sunflower oil, wheat germ, fish oil, mixed vegetable oil, linseed oil and walnut oil. They are usually liquid at room temperature, but will solidify in a fridge.

Heating polyunsaturated oil makes it toxic, so these oils should preferably be cold-pressed, stored in a fridge and eaten uncooked. It is easy to add a small amount each day to salads, cooked vegetables or spread on bread. These are high in omega-3 and omega-6 essential fatty acids (see earlier).

Monounsaturated Fats (MUFAs)

Olive oil, hazelnut oil, peanut oil, rapeseed oil, almond oil are rich in these types of fats. Monounsaturated fats contain oleic acid (omega-9 fatty acids) that helps to keep arteries supple. These fats are more stable with heat and so are preferred for cooking.

Trans Fatty Acids And Hydrogenation

Trans fatty acids are unsaturated fatty acids with an unusual shape, so the body treats them more like saturated fatty acids. Dairy products, lamb and beef contain small amounts of trans fatty acids. When vegetable oils are artificially hardened to produce margarine trans fatty acids are produced. Trans fats are most commonly found in biscuits, cakes, pastries (savoury and sweet), sausages, crackers and take-away food. High intake of trans fatty acids has been linked to heart disease. Because the trans fatty acids are difficult for the body to metabolise, they accumulate in blood vessels causing blockages. Trans fatty acids can also interfere with the metabolism of essential fatty acids. Some studies suggest that trans fats are worse than saturated fats for health.

Food manufacturers want a solid fat that does not go rancid easily and does not have any real taste, but vegetable oil is liquid at room temperature. Hydrogenation gives them this.

Hydrogenation is a high tech process. Vegetable seeds are cleaned and bleached to remove all colour, taste, smells and impurities. The liquid vegetable oil is then heated to high temperatures and a catalyst (commonly nickel, but could be palladium, platinum or rhodium) is added. Hydrogen is bubbled through the liquid. The mixture is then filtered to remove the metal, leaving hydrogenated vegetable oil. Water, whey, salt, vitamins, colourings, flavourings and emulsifiers may then be added to produce hydrogenated margarine.

The advantage of all this is that it gives a uniform product that is solid at room temperature and has a long shelf life. This last characteristic is very important both for manufacturers and consumers. It gives manufacturers increased flexibility, and it means that consumers can buy products and not have to worry so much about 'best before' dates. This seems like a win-win situation for everyone, but there is a potential problem: the hydrogenation process changes some of the fats into trans fatty acids.

It is easy to blame the manufacturer, but as long as we, the consumers, prefer to buy long-shelf life products that always taste and look the same, manufacturers will continue to produce them using hydrogenated fats.

Frying, particularly at high temperatures, also produces trans fatty acids.

Summary Of The Advantages And Disadvantages Of Different Types Of Fats

	Advantages	Disadvantages
Saturated	Stable under heat	Converted into cholesterol
Polyunsaturated	Contains EFAs	Unstable under heat
Monounsaturated	Stable under heat; keep arteries supple	No EFAs
Trans fatty acids		Linked to heart disease; no EFAs; interfere with EFA metabolism

Custom Blends Of Oils

Using muscle testing it is possible to work out a custom blend of oil for a client. Test:

- How many oils to use

- Which oils – we have a list of 33 different oils to choose from.

- Anything special about the oils, e.g. possibilities include that the oils must be a certain brand, must be cold pressed or must be organic.

- What proportions for each oil, e.g. 2 parts of olive oil, 3 parts of walnut oil, 1 x 500 mg EPO capsule, etc.

- What the dose is, how it is to be taken (frequency, time of day, with other food, etc.). Sometimes the oil blend would be suitable to use in cooking, put on cooked food or use as a salad dressing, but it is important to test that these options are suitable.

- Are there any constraints on how far in advance the mixture can be made up.

- How long to be taken or when do you retest.

Oils that could be used include:

1. Almond oil
2. Avocado oil
3. Blackcurrant seed oil - supplement
4. Butter
5. Castor oil
6. Coconut oil
7. Corn oil
8. Cottonseed oil
9. Evening primrose oil - supplement

10. Fish oil
11. Grape seed oil
12. Hazelnut oil
13. Hemp oil - supplement
14. Lard
15. Linseed (flaxseed) oil - supplement
16. Macadamia oil
17. Mustard oil (available in the UK from shops selling Indian spices, etc.)
18. Olive oil
19. Palm oil
20. Peanut oil
21. Pecan oil
22. Perilla oil – used in Korean cuisine
23. Pumpkin seed oil
24. Rape seed / Canola oil
25. Safflower oil
26. Sea buckthorn oil - supplement
27. Sesame oil
28. Soya oil
29. Starflower (borage) oil - supplement
30. Sunflower oil
31. Sweet almond oil
32. Walnut oil
33. Wheat germ oil

So testing might look like this:

Are we looking for a custom oil blend for Kate? Yes
How many oils are we using – at least 3? Yes
More than 3? No
So, three oils? Yes [confirming question]
Are any of the oils in the first 10 on the list? Yes
Number 1 to 5 inclusive? Yes
Almond? No
Avocado? No
Blackcurrant? Yes
Are any of the other oils in the first 10 on the list? Yes
[Find the rest of the oils]
So the blend is blackcurrant, olive and walnut oils – is that correct? Yes
Do we need to know any more about the oils themselves? No
For the blackcurrant oil how many parts – more than 1? No
[Find the number of parts for each oil]
So, it is 1 part blackcurrant, 2 parts olive oil and 1 part walnut oil, is that correct? Yes
[confirmation question]
So the dose is more than a teaspoonful at a time? Yes
More than two teaspoonfuls? No

Two teaspoonfuls? No
1 and a half teaspoonfuls? Yes
[Continue testing to find the rest of the information, such as how often the dose it taken, any special requirements or restrictions and for how long.]

Butter Versus Margarine

Clients may ask you whether they should use butter or margarine. The facts are that butter is loaded with saturated fat, and almost all margarines have some saturated fat and, more significantly, trans fatty acids. Testing may indicate a preference for one or the other, or a reduction in both.

Problems With A High Fat Diet

- Increased risk of obesity (supplies 9 calories per gram of fat compared with 4 calories per gram of carbohydrate)

- Increased risk of cancer (breast, colon and prostate)

- Increased risk of heart problems (high blood pressure, heart disease)

- Gall bladder disease

- Insulin resistance

- High fat diets line the stomach with lipids and stop the absorption of antioxidants.

Problems With A Low Fat Diet

Some vitamins are fat-soluble and so are found in foods that contain fat. They also need fat for transportation into the body. Essential fatty acids are, as their name implies, essential for health.

A study published in the *American Journal of Epidemiology* in 2007 (Park S, Murphy SP, Wilkens LR, et al. *Calcium, vitamin D, and dairy product intake and prostate cancer risk: the Multiethnic Cohort Study* 2007;166:1259-1269) showed a positive correlation between low-fat and non-fat milk consumption and the risk of prostate cancer. This link was not there for whole milk.

Cholesterol (14)

On the menu we have:

14 **Cholesterol Levels**
  ➤ Reduce intake of cholesterol rich foods
  ➤ Reduce saturated fat intake (see page 82)
  ➤ Increase fibre (see page 69)
  ➤ Increase nutrient(s) involved in homocysteine metabolism
  ➤ Increase consumption of stanols and sterols
      ＊ From food
      ＊ From functional food products

Cholesterol is a waxy type of fat, found in animal products (meat, dairy products and eggs). The body makes its own cholesterol in the liver from saturated fats. Cholesterol is essential for good health, as it is used:

- To make bile acids, skin, steroid hormones and myelin around nerves.

- To stabilise cell membranes.

Types Of Cholesterol
Cholesterol joins with lipoproteins in order to travel around the body. There are two types of cholesterol:

- LDL Cholesterol (low density lipoprotein cholesterol), also known as 'bad' cholesterol.

- HDL Cholesterol (high density lipoprotein cholesterol), also known as good cholesterol.

People are often tested these days for cholesterol levels, but it is important that they are also tested for the proportions of HDL and LDL cholesterol.

LDL Cholesterol
High blood levels of cholesterol in the form of low-density lipoproteins are linked with narrowing of the arteries (atherosclerosis) and coronary artery disease.
LDL cholesterol molecules are small enough to seep into artery walls and fur them up. Deposits of cholesterol along artery walls can block blood flow, both directly and by making the arteries

less flexible. A severe blockage can result in a heart attack or angina.

People who are overweight and/or do not take any exercise are more likely to have high LDL cholesterol levels. People with poorly controlled diabetes, low thyroid levels, or some liver and kidney diseases may also have high levels of LDL. Some drugs such as beta blockers and steroids can affect blood cholesterol levels. High cholesterol levels can also run in families.

HDL Cholesterol

Cholesterol in the blood in the form of high-density lipoproteins seems to protect against arterial disease. HDL's are mainly taking cholesterol to the liver for excretion, whereas LDL's are taking cholesterol to the tissues.

Cholesterol And Diet

Liver, kidneys, eggs and prawns are higher in dietary cholesterol than other foods. Some years ago the medical profession placed a lot of emphasis on reducing cholesterol in the diet, but current research suggests that has less impact on lowering bad cholesterol in the body than previously thought.

Saturated fat in the diet is changed into LDL-cholesterol (see page 87). Reducing saturated fat intake can have a direct effect on cholesterol levels.

Cholesterol is broken down into bile acids and excreted via the stools. A high fibre diet helps this process as the dietary fibre binds with bile acids and speeds their transit through the gut. If bile acids are not removed from the gut, they are reabsorbed and eventually re-converted into cholesterol.

Homocysteine And Co-Factors

Recently interest has focussed on homocysteine. It is an amino acid formed as a breakdown product of another amino acid, methionine. When a body is well nourished, homocysteine is converted into other harmless compounds. The nutrients involved in this process are vitamins B6, B12 and folic acid. When these nutrients are not readily available, elevated blood levels of homocysteine result, leading to arterial lesions. This starts a chain reaction ending in atherosclerosis, the major precursor of heart disease.

Stanols And Sterols

Plant stanols and sterols occur naturally in foods such as fruits, vegetables, nuts, seeds, cereals, legumes, olive and peanut oils. It is thought that people generally consume about 150-400mg per day of naturally occurring stanols and sterols. This level is too low to have any significant effect on cholesterol levels.

An interest has grown in adding these to foods and so creating functional foods that lower cholesterol. The stanols and sterols are modified slightly to make this possible. Typical foods include yoghurt drinks and spreads.

Stanols and sterols work by reducing cholesterol absorption in the intestine. The British Dietetic Association says: "2-3g per day is the amount that research has shown to give an effect in people with raised cholesterol levels."

Stanols and sterols used in this way may lower cholesterol, but some see this as an artificial way of reducing cholesterol with uncertainty about the long-term effects.

Vitamins (15)

(Information on individual vitamins is in appendix A1.)

On the menu we have:

15 Vitamins
- ➤ Increase
  - * Through food
  - * Through supplementation
- ➤ Decrease
  - * Through food
  - * Through supplementation

Functions Of Vitamins

Vitamins are organic substances that we need in small amounts to perform various physiological functions. Vitamins are essential for normal growth and development, and are involved in many chemical reactions in the body. Functions include:

- Helping the body use the calories in food.

- Helping process proteins, carbohydrates and fats.

- Involved in building cells, tissues and organs.

- Some vitamins work as antioxidants. (See page 99)

Essential Vitamins

There are known to be 13 essential vitamins. They are:

- Vitamin A

- Vitamin C

- Vitamin D

- Vitamin E

- Vitamin K

- Vitamin B1 (thiamine)

- Vitamin B2 (riboflavin)

- Vitamin B3 (niacin)

- Vitamin B5 (pantothenic acid)

- Biotin

- Vitamin B6

- Vitamin B12

- Folate (folic acid)

Types Of Vitamins

Vitamins can be:

- Fat-soluble: vitamins A, D, E and K
  Absorbed along with fats in the small intestine.
  Excess stored in the body's fatty tissue particularly the liver.
  Supplements best taken with meals.

- Water-soluble: B vitamins and vitamin C
  Absorbed by diffusion along with water and dissolve in body fluids.
  Must be used by the body right away.
  Any left over water-soluble vitamins leave the body through the urine.
  Supplements can be taken with or away from meals.

Vitamins Made In the Body

The body can make some vitamins:

- Vitamin K and some B vitamins in the large intestine.

- Vitamin D from the action of sunlight on the skin.

- Vitamin A from the provitamin carotene.

Vitamin Deficiencies

Vitamin deficiencies can come about because:

- There is not enough of the vitamin in the diet.

- The body has an increased need for the vitamin because of lifestyle, interaction with drugs (see Appendix D2) or medical considerations.

- Inability to process the vitamins in the food. This may be because of general digestive problems, or relate to a specific vitamin.

- Individual has a particularly high need for that vitamin.

Food And Vitamin Content
The vitamin content can vary:

- Fruit and vegetables have their highest level of vitamins when they are picked ripe.

- Eating foods immediately after picking ensures maximum vitamin intake.

- Water-soluble vitamins tend to be light sensitive so store fruit and vegetables in a dark place.

- Warmth can degrade some vitamins, so store in a cool place or frozen.

- Cooking may destroy vitamins (but see page 110).

- Using large amounts of water for cooking vegetables and then throwing the water away reduces the amount of water-soluble vitamins in the food.

- Fruit and vegetables that have been frozen while fresh may contain more nutrients than ones that have been stored in a fridge or at ambient temperature.

Toxic Effects Of Vitamins
More is not always better.   High doses of certain vitamins can be poisonous. This is particularly true of the fat-soluble vitamins (see page 142, 155 and 157) that are stored in the liver. See under individual vitamins for more information.

Official Recommendations
Most governments have recommendations for vitamin intake from food and/or supplements, but these vary from country to country. Measures include:

- Recommended dietary allowances (RDAs): the recommended daily allowances to prevent deficiency.

- Reference nutrient intake (RNI): the daily amount estimated to be sufficient for 97% of a specified population group.

- Upper Safe Limit (USL) is the maximum amount to eat or take as a supplement without the risk of side effects from poisoning. These limits can be different for short and long term use.

Testing For Vitamins

Usually testing will relate to one particular vitamin. The client may need to increase or decrease it. The change can relate to food content or supplementation or both. Sometimes it is not important to the body how the increase happens, as long as it does happen. In these cases ask the clients whether they would prefer to increase food intake or take a supplement, and then test accordingly.

If the increase is going to be through food, you need to check that the client does not have any problem with those foods (e.g. allergy). See the section on Avoidance, Replacements, Reductions And Additions (page 19).

For a detailed discussion of supplements turn to page 132.

(Information on individual vitamins is in Appendix A1.)

Minerals (16)

(Information on individual minerals is in Appendix A2)

On the menu we have:

16 Minerals
- ➤ Increase
    - * Through food
    - * Through supplementation
- ➤ Decrease
    - * Through food
    - * Through supplementation

Mineral Content Of the Body

Minerals constitute about 4% of body weight mainly in the skeleton. If the human body were left to decompose completely then approximately 5 pounds of elemental mineral ash would be left:

- 75% would be calcium and phosphorus

- Approximately one teaspoon of iron

- Approximately two teaspoons of salt (sodium chloride)

- Over two teaspoons of potassium

- The rest would be many other minerals

(Information source: Elson M Haas)

Types Of Minerals

Minerals needed by human beings are divided into:

- Macro-minerals: minerals of which the body needs at least 100 mg per day; e.g. calcium, phosphorus, sodium chloride, magnesium, iron, etc.

- Trace minerals or micro-minerals: the body needs less of these; e.g. zinc, selenium, chromium.

Some minerals – arsenic, aluminium, silicon and nickel – are present in the body but their function is not known.

Minerals, in general, do not exist in a pure form, but occur as salts (e.g. sodium chloride).

Function Of Minerals
Minerals have three general functions in the body:

- Enzymes need minerals such as calcium, iron and zinc in order to carry out their function.

- The electrolyte minerals (sodium and potassium chloride) are used by cells to carry electrical impulses (nerve impulses and muscle contractions) in the body fluids through the cells and to other cells.

- They are a basic part of all cell structures.

- Minerals are used to build bones and teeth. Zinc provides structural integrity to proteins important for DNA transcription.

Absorption Of Minerals
Phytic acid (see page 70), tannins (from tea, wine, pomegranates, etc.) and oxalates inhibit the absorption of many minerals. Minerals with similar charges often compete for the same intestinal transport protein, so taking excess of one can lead to a deficiency (through lack of absorption) of another.

Acid foods and supplements such as vitamin C enhance absorption.

Amino acid chelates (AAC) are minerals that are organically bound to amino acids. This process occurs naturally in the body and can also be carried out in the laboratory. This chelating process is often used in supplements as it can enhance the absorption of the mineral.

For official recommendations and testing for minerals see vitamins (page 92 onwards).

(Information on individual minerals is in Appendix A2)

Phytochemicals (17)

On the menu we have:

17 Phytochemicals
- ➤ Increase
  - * In general
  - * Specific food(s)
  - * Supplements
- ➤ {Decrease} – **unlikely**
  - * See under increase phytochemicals

The terms phytonutrients and phytochemicals are used interchangeably. 'Phyto' is from the Greek word meaning plants.

Phytochemicals are not essential nutrients but are substances in food that have been found to enhance health, e.g. reduce the risk of certain cancers and cardiovascular disease, and of age-related blindness. Many phytochemicals are also antioxidants (see page 99).

Well over 100 of these substances have been identified and many of them seem to have an important effect in supporting the endocrine and immune systems.

Good Sources Of Phytochemicals
Plentiful supplies of phytochemicals are found in fruit and vegetables, but some seem to be particularly good sources of these nutrients including:

- Apples

- Beans and peas

- Berries

- Buckwheat

- Blueberries

- Mustard Family – including broccoli, Brussels sprouts and cauliflower (see page 179)

- Chilli

- Citrus fruit

- Dark green leafy vegetables

- Flax seeds and oil (see also page 79)

- Garlic

- Tea (but see page 118)

- Herbs and spices

- Nuts

- Onions

- Seeds

- Soya Beans and tofu

- Tomatoes

- Whole grains

- Wine (but see page 116)

Testing for phytochemicals might look like this:

> *So, we are looking at phytochemicals – is that correct?* Yes
> *Does Tom need to increase his phytochemical intake generally?* No
> *Are we looking for one particular food?* Yes [Note that it could be more than one food.]
> *Is it on the list?* Yes [If you got 'no' to this questions, read page 17 on finding foods.]
> *Is it from here to here?* Yes [Touching the list in two places.]
> *From here to here?* No [First half of the part in last question.]
> *From here to here?* Yes [Second half of the part in last question.]
> This one? No
> *This one?* Yes
> *So, is it the cabbage family?* Yes [Check question.]
> *Is it a specific member of the cabbage family?* No
> *Is it the cabbage family in general?* Yes [A check question that also establishes that it is not 2 or more members of the cabbage family.]
> *So, Tom needs to increase the amount of the cabbage family in* his diet – is that correct?
> Yes
> [Then you would find out by how much, etc.]

Antioxidants And Free Radicals (18)

On the menu we have:

18 Antioxidants
> Increase
* In general
* Foods
– Anti-oxidant groups
– Specific food
* Supplements
> {Decrease} - **unlikely**
* As under increase

Free Radicals

Free radicals are a natural by-product of metabolic processes when oxygen combines with food to produce energy (ATP).

Free radicals:

- Destroy harmful bacteria.

- Fight inflammation.

- Maintain smooth muscle tone.

Free radicals are unstable and seek out electrons from other molecules, particularly hydrogen. Other molecules break down when the free radicals "steal" electrons from them.

Free radical production is a natural and normal part of the body's activities. Free radicals perform some useful functions in the body, and the body has ways of neutralising the excess.

Problems occur if the excess exceeds the body's capacity to deal with it. An excess of free radicals can be caused by:

- Smoking

- Sunbathing

- Frying food

- Infections
- Excessive exercise
- Stress
- Radiation
- Polluted environments

Excess free radicals are a problem because they attack the body itself, damaging key cellular molecules such as DNA. When the cell membrane is oxidised it is either hardened so that nutrients cannot get into the cell, or it may be punctured so that the cell collapses as the cell fluid drains out. In the skin this leads to skin which is leathery or wrinkled and sagging; in the joints this causes the synovial fluid to lose its lubricating quality, in cells it may damage the DNA causing inappropriate cell division and the possibility of cancer, etc. Cells with damaged DNA may be more prone to developing cancer. Free radical activity has also been implicated in premature ageing, heart disease, arthritis, cataract formation, chronic fatigue syndrome, etc.

Under normal circumstances antioxidant enzymes and nutrients deactivate these superfluous free radicals.

Antioxidants

Anti-oxidants provide the free radicals with the additional electron they seek without becoming damaged in the process. Our bodies produce anti-oxidants, but may need additional anti-oxidants either in food or as a supplement to combat free-radical damage. This is particularly true now because the environment has become so polluted.

The main anti-oxidants groups are:

- Beta-carotene: the plant source of vitamin A found in fruit and vegetables
- Vitamins C & E
- Bioflavonoids from citrus fruit
- Pycnogenols (also known as proanthocyanidins) from white and maritime pine bark, seeds and skin of red grapes
- Curcuminoids from turmeric, mustard, corn and yellow peppers
- Lutein from fruit and vegetables (particularly kale, spinach, lettuce, parsley and broccoli)
- Lycopene from tomatoes, pink grapefruit, guava and water melon
- Zeanxanthin from corn, spinach, cabbage, broccoli, peas and chicory leaf
- Digestive enzymes amylase and protease which are produced by the body and found in many foods, but are destroyed by cooking

- Antioxidant enzymes glutathione peroxidase and catalase are produced by the body and found in apples, grapes, mango, mushrooms and honey. They help combat hydrogen peroxide, which is produced in the body as a metabolic by-product, and decomposes into free radicals. Selenium is needed for the body to manufacture glutathione peroxidase

- Zinc and manganese are needed to form antioxidant superoxide dismutase which combats the superoxide radical

- Ginkgo biloba – taken as a supplement – it is able to cross the blood-brain barrier, which is a network of blood vessels with closely spaced cells that makes it difficult for potentially toxic substances to penetrate the blood vessel walls and enter the brain.

Uric acid and bilirubin (produced from the breakdown of haem – the red iron-containing pigment found in haemoglobin) are anti-oxidants produced by the body.

Ideally people should eat/take a full range of anti-oxidants because:

- Some anti-oxidants are water-soluble and some are fat-soluble; the ones that are water-soluble are effective in the watery parts of the body; the ones that are fat-soluble are effective in fatty tissues such as cell membranes. (Pycnogenols are unusual in that they are effective in fatty and watery tissues.)

- Some anti-oxidants work synergistically with others (e.g. vitamins A and E).

- Some work in specific areas (e.g. vitamin A and beta carotene work in the cell membrane; vitamin E works on the surface of the cells; vitamin C can work inside and outside the cell membrane).

- Some have large molecules that cannot get through the gut wall (e.g. pine bark) and so are protective within the intestine (counteract chemicals in food, protective against colon cancer and intestinal polyps).

Prebiotics And Probiotics (19)

On the menu we have:

19 Prebiotics And Probiotics
  - ➤ Increase prebiotics
    - ✳ Food
    - ✳ Supplement
  - ➤ Decrease prebiotics
    - ✳ Food
    - ✳ Supplement
  - ➤ Increase Probiotics
    - ✳ Food
    - ✳ Supplement
  - ➤ Decrease Probiotics
    - ✳ Food
    - ✳ Supplement

A Healthy Gut

The gut contains billions of friendly bacteria. It is estimated that there are about 500 different ones. About 60% of faeces are made up of bacteria.

The bacteria are very useful for our health:

- They produce biotin (a B vitamin) and vitamin K.

- They protect against colon cancer.

- They are involved in the immune system response of the body.

- They ferment unused food.

- They are involved in lowering blood cholesterol levels.

- They prevent the growth of organisms that could cause food poisoning.

Stress, antibiotics, certain drugs and female hormones can cause the balance to tip away from the favourable bacteria and towards unfavourable organisms.

Probiotics

The FAO/WHO define probiotics as: 'Live micro-organisms which when administered in adequate amounts confer a health benefit on the host'. The beneficial bacteria in the gut help to keep harmful bacteria in check. Probiotics provide these beneficial bacteria. The main difficulty with increasing healthy bacteria by taking them orally is that many are destroyed by the stomach acid. Certain strains, such as Lactobacillus acidophilus La-5 and Bifidobacterium have been shown to have the best chance of surviving.

Not all strains of bacteria have a probiotic effect. For example, Lactobacillus bulgaricus and Streptococcus thermophilus (used to make yoghurt) do not have this effect.

Prebiotics

Prebiotics are food for the healthy gut bacteria. These are mainly soluble fibre that cannot be broken down by the body's own enzymes, so pass unaltered into the colon. In the colon they act as food for the probiotic bacteria, so helping to increase the number of friendly ones. Prebiotics include inulin and oligosaccharides. Fructo-oligosaccardies (FOS) is the type that the research has been done on. Both inulin and FOS can be taken as nutritional supplements (see page 132).

The main food sources are onions, leeks, garlic, Jerusalem artichoke, wild yam, asparagus, chicory root, oats, and unrefined wheat and barley. It may be difficult to eat sufficient of these to have a meaningful impact on gut flora, so taking supplements is often preferred.

Increasing the prebiotic content of the diet either through food or supplements can initially lead to flatulence and gas, so it may be advisable to start with a lower dose at first, and build up the intake as the population of friendly bacteria increases.

Testing For Prebiotics And Probiotics

There are a very limited number of probiotic foods – live yoghurt, kaffir and manufactured probiotic drinks are the obvious choices. Probiotic drinks are often very high in sugar and for this reason may not be appropriate.

There are many probiotic supplements available. See the Supplement section (page 132) for more detailed information on testing supplements.

Probiotics can be bought as supplements in their own right or in a supplement with probiotics.

Food Combining (20)

On the menu we have:

20   Food Combining / Uncombining
  - ➤ Standard food combining advice
  - ➤ Standard food combining advice with variations
  - ➤   Combining foods
    - *   Food category with food category
    - *   Specific food with particular food
    - *   Specific food with a category of food
  - ➤ Uncombining foods
    - *   As above
  - ➤ Other

The less healthy a client is the more likely it is that they will benefit from practising food combining. As a person becomes healthier they are able to tolerate a larger range of foods and more different combinations of food. (See page 5.)

In practical terms some people benefit from eating many small meals made up of one food at a time rather than trying to have a few meals that combine several categories of foods.

Standard Food Combining Theory

Mainstream scientific understanding does not support the food combining theory, but this does not mean that the theory is necessarily wrong. This approach to diet was popularised by Doris Grant and Jean Joice in their book *Food Combining for Health*. The main elements of it are:

  - ■   Proteins need an acid medium for digestion.

  - ■   Carbohydrates (starches and sugars) require an alkaline medium.

  - ■   When a meal contains both types of foods, there is too much acid in the stomach for carbohydrate digestion and not enough for protein digestion.

  - ■   If fruit is eaten with other foods, their digestion is delayed and fermentation may result.

  - ■   Fruits are divided into three classes: acid, sub-acid and sweet.

Standard Food Combining Advice

The main elements of the advice are:

- Carbohydrate and proteins are eaten separately.

- Carbohydrates can be eaten with vegetables.

- Proteins can be eaten with vegetables.

- Fruit is eaten on its own or with other fruits from the same class (acid, sub-acid or sweet).

- Melon is usually eaten alone.

- Pulses are only eaten sprouted.

Criticism Of Food Combining

There are various criticisms of food combining:

- Medical and conventionally trained nutritionists argue that there is no physiological reason why protein and carbohydrate cannot be absorbed at the same meal.

- Some food naturally contains proteins and carbohydrates, e.g. pulses.

- Many classic food dishes contain combinations that break food combining rules, e.g. apple pie, bread and cheese, etc.

- Benefits people experience could be because they have changed what they are eating as the diet has made them more aware.

Testing For Food Combining

If food combining comes up, the easiest way to proceed is to first find out if the client is going to be following the standard food combining advice either in its entirety or with minor variations. So testing might look like this:

> *Are we looking at food combining?* Yes
> *Is it appropriate for Meg to follow the standard food combining advice in its entirety?* No
> *Is the standard food combining advice a good place to start?* Yes
> *So should Meg eat carbohydrate and protein separately?* Yes
> [Work out how far apart they need to be.]
> *Is it appropriate to eat carbohydrate with vegetables?* Yes
> *Is it appropriate to eat protein with vegetables?* No
> *So, if Meg eats protein, how long must she wait before she eats vegetables? More than a hour?* Yes
> [Etc.]

But sometimes the standard food combining is not a good place to start:

Are we looking at food combining? Yes
Is it appropriate for Ronald to follow the standard food combining advice in its entirety? No
Is the standard food combining advice a good place to start? No

This probably means that you need to be looking for two items that the client should put together (aids digestion or absorption) or should keep apart (consuming together causes problem). Food combining may increase tolerance to various foods, e.g. adding a slice of lemon to tap water will often increase tolerance to the tap water. Inappropriate food combining will reduce tolerance to the foods involved. The questioning continues:

Are we looking at combining foods? No
Uncombining foods? Yes

Whether you got a positive response to putting foods together or keeping them apart, you now need to establish whether you are looking for categories or individual foods; there are three possibilities:

- Combining/Uncombining category A and category B (e.g. dairy with the deadly nightshade family)
- Combining/Uncombining food A and food B (e.g. orange and milk)
- Combining/Uncombining category A and food B (e.g. dairy products and onions)

So the questioning might carry on from the last lot of questioning like this:

Are we looking for two categories? No
Are we looking for two separate foods? No
Are we looking for a category and a separate food? Yes

Page 17 gives guidance on how then to narrow down to the exact category and individual food.

Occasionally two foods put together may be fine, but adding a third may cause problems, e.g. it is possible that A+B is O.K., A+C is O.K., B+C is O.K. but A+B+C is not O.K. In this case, the questioning would look like this:

Are we looking for two categories? No
Are we looking for two separate foods? No
Are we looking for a category and a separate food? No
So, is this more than 2 categories/groups? Yes
[Etc.]

How Far Apart?

It is not enough to establish that a client should not eat two foods or categories of foods at the same time; it is important to establish how far apart they should be, but the time may vary depending which one is eaten first. If the client eats A before B may have to wait a different length of time than if eat B before A. Testing might look like this:

So should Thomas eat A and B separately? Yes
So if Thomas eats A, how long must he wait before he eats B – more than 1 hour? Yes
More than 2 hours? Yes
More than 3 hours? No
So, between 2 and 3 hours? Yes
Do we need to be more precise? Yes
[Narrow down to find the exact time window.]
If Thomas eats B first does he need to wait the same amount of time before eating A? No
Is it less? Yes
[Etc.]

This makes sense because digestion of A may take longer than digestion of B.

Acid/Alkaline Balance (21)

On the menu we have:

21 Acid Alkaline Balance
- ➤ {Decreasing alkaline forming foods} - **unlikely**
- ➤ Decreasing acid forming foods
  - ✳ Overall
  - ✳ Particular food type
- ➤ Increasing alkaline forming foods
  - ✳ Overall
  - ✳ Particular food type
- ➤ {Increasing acid forming foods} - **unlikely**

"We humans have a problem: we are alkaline by design and acid by function" Enzyme Pro News October 1999

Acidity And pH

Acidity or alkalinity of substances is measured by their pH (potential of Hydrogen). The scale is 0-14 where 14 is alkaline. A score of 7 is neutral. Each point on the scale represents an increase of 10 times, e.g. a pH of 9 is 10 times more alkaline than a pH of 8.

A pH range of 7.4 to 7.5 is regarded as associated with good health.

When a food is metabolised a mineral ash is formed:

- Alkaline foods: the ash is rich in calcium, magnesium, sodium and potassium.

- Acid foods: the ash is rich in chlorine, phosphorus and sulphur.

When acid foods are metabolised acids are produced which are neutralised by calcium carbonate, magnesium carbonate, potassium carbonate and sodium carbonate. So from a dietary point of view the more acid foods you eat, the more minerals you need from alkaline foods to neutralise them.

Acid Alkaline Balance

The overall acid/alkaline balance of the body is affected by:

- The type of food we eat – the more acid food the more stress is placed on the body to maintain the correct pH.

- Intake of the alkaline salts (in food or supplements).

- Levels of stress

- Exercise levels

- Excess alcohol

In the short term the body is able to buffer any excess acid via alkaline reserves in the blood and bones, but a long-term acid diet results in this buffering capacity becoming exhausted. This means that a high protein intake can lead, for example, to bone-density loss, as the calcium is taken out of the bones to neutralise the excess acidity, and so can lead to osteoporosis.

Alkaline Forming Food

In general most writers in this field seem to agree on the following:

- Vegetables, including potatoes cooked in their skins.

- Salad.

- Fresh fruit including citrus fruit (except plums and cranberries).

- Almonds.

- Milk is mildly alkaline-forming.

Acid Forming Food

In general most writers seem to agree on the following:

- Animal proteins.

- Nuts (except almonds).

- Starchy foods.

- Sugar.

- Plums and cranberries.

Although we think of citrus fruit as acid foods, the end result of their metabolism is alkaline ash, so they are included in the alkaline foods group. The general recommendation is to eat a diet consisting of 80% alkali-forming foods.

Symptoms Of Excess Acidity

There are many symptoms associated with excess acidity, but, of course, these symptoms could be caused or exacerbated by other factors.

Symptoms include irritability, pessimism, restless sleep patterns, waking tired, aches and pains, shortness of breath, indigestion and cravings. Excess acidity is also thought to contribute to the development of diabetes, arthritis etc.

Testing For Acid Alkaline Balance

In one sense reducing acid forming foods is the same thing as increasing alkaline forming foods, unless the total amount eaten is being increased. Testing may show a preference for expressing it one way or the other. If it does not matter which way it is done, you will get a 'yes' to reducing acid foods or a 'yes' to increasing alkaline foods, depending on which one you ask about first.

Testing might look like this:

> *Are we looking at acid alkaline balance?* Yes
> *Does Sam need to decrease acid forming foods?* No
> *Does Sam need to increase alkaline forming foods?* Yes
> *Is this all alkaline forming food?* No
> *Is it one specific food or food group?* Yes
> *Is it a food group?* No
> *Is it a vegetable?* Yes
> [Etc.]

Raw And Cooked Food (22)

On the menu we have:

22 Raw/ Cooked Foods
- ➤ Decreasing raw foods
  - * All
  - * Category of foods
  - * Specific food (s)
- ➤ Increasing raw food
  - * As above
- ➤ Decreasing cooked foods
  - * As above
- ➤ Increasing cooked food
  - * As above

Reasons For Eating Foods Raw

There are many sound nutritional and physiological reasons for eating food raw:

- Humans have evolved to eat raw foods.

- Cooking destroys some nutrients, particularly vitamins B and C.

- Cooking changes some nutrients into harmful foods, e.g. polyunsaturates become trans fatty acids. (See page 83)

- Raw foods contain digestive enzymes (mainly amylase and protease) that aid digestion.

- Cooked food is 'dead' food, as cooking destroys the living cells.

- Too much cooked food has been linked to a lowering of the immune function in the body.

Reasons For Eating Food Cooked

It is often assumed that it is better to eat food raw, but there are also compelling reasons for eating food cooked.

- Cooking breaks down cell walls and makes some nutrients more available for digestion, e.g. 3-4% of carotenoids absorbed from raw food, but 15-20% absorbed from cooked food.

- Cooking can make food less bulky to eat. (Juicing also does, and does not have some of the drawbacks of cooked food.)

- Cooking destroys harmful organisms (e.g. salmonella) in meat etc.

- Cooking destroys harmful substances in some foods, e.g. trypsin-inhibitors in raw pulses block the action of the enzyme trypsin; sprouting or cooking the pulse destroys this.

- Some people appear to tolerate some foods better if the food is cooked, e.g. eggs

Oriental Medicine

Oriental medicine advises a predominantly raw food diet for those suffering from hot, inflammatory conditions, but not for those suffering from muscular weakness, severe fatigue, fluid retention or cold conditions.

Possible Raw Foods

There are many possible raw foods. In testing you could be looking to increase (or decrease) a particular group (e.g. nuts and seeds) or a particular food (e.g. raw carrots). Here is a list of possible raw foods:

- Fruit

- Vegetables

- Herbs

- Spices

- Flowers

- Sprouted pulses and sprouted grains

- Nuts and seeds

- Cold pressed oil

- Eggs

- Fish

- Raw milk

Processed Foods (23)

On the menu we have:

23 Processed Foods
- ➤ Decrease processed food
  - ∗ Group of foods
  - ∗ Specific food
- ➤ {Increase} processed food - **unlikely**

Health Issues With Processed Foods
Processed food tends to be:

- High in saturated fats (see page 82).

- High in trans fatty acids (see page 83).

- High in salt and/or sugar (see page 119).

- High in food additives (see page 114).

- Low in nutrients.

- Low in fibre (see page 69).

Testing For Processed Foods
Often the quickest way to find which processed foods are involved is by asking the person which processed foods they eat. This includes at home and while 'on the go', so testing might look like this:

Is the next area we look at processed foods? Yes
So, does Allan need to reduce his processed food intake? Yes
Is it all processed food? No [This may seem surprising, but it may be because the client would find it so difficult to stop all processed food that they would do nothing.]
[Ask Allan what processed food he eats. He says he has burgers and French fries once a week, and gets a cake from the bakery near his office if he knows he is going to be working late.]
So, is it the burger and fries we need to look at? No [Notice have used the phrase 'look at' rather than 'stop' as this is more general.]

Is it the cake he eats when working late? Yes
Is it to stop completely? Yes

It is important to ask the person what they would use as replacement and check out that that is not a problem too. (See page 19.)

Food Additives (24)

On the menu we have:

24 Food Additives
- ➤ Decrease/stop food additive(s)
  - * Individual additive
  - * Particular category
- ➤ {Increase food additives} - **unlikely**

What Are Food Additives?

Food additives are chemicals that are added to food to enhance colour, flavour and keeping qualities or to facilitate processing.

Many people are allergic to additives in food (see page 114). Additives can be added to heighten the flavour, so that low-nutrient foods can taste more palatable. Often the lack of real ingredients is disguised by resorting to artificial flavourings and colourings.

Some people also react to natural food colourings (e.g. E162, Betanin from beetroot). Sometimes this is because they are allergic to the actual substance, but more often it is because of the solvents that are used for their extraction. Solvents etc. are not required to be named in the list of ingredients because they are part of the processing and not intended to be part of the finished product, although minute traces will remain.

Categories Of Food Additives

Food additives can be divided into several groups, but some chemicals would occur in more than one group as they perform more than one function. Although food additives are put into categories like this, it is unusual for a person to have a problem with the whole category. It is much more likely to be one or two chemicals.

Name	Function	Examples
Acids	Make flavours "sharper", and also act as preservatives and antioxidants	Vinegar, citric acid, tartaric acid, malic acid, lactic acid.
Acidity Regulators	Change or otherwise control the acidity and alkalinity of foods.	Acetic acid, potassium lactate, citric acid
Anti-caking Agents	Keep powders such as milk powder from caking or sticking.	Calcium carbonate, magnesium oxide, silicon dioxide
Antifoaming Agents	Reduce or prevent foaming in foods.	Dimethylpolysiloxane oxystearin
Antioxidants	Inhibit the effects of oxygen on food.	Vitamin C, sulphur dioxide, lecithin
Bulking Agents	Increase the bulk of a food without increasing its nutritional value.	Starch
Food Colouring	Replace colours lost during preparation, or to make food look more attractive.	Tartrazine (E102) and annatto (E160b)
Colour Retention Agents	Preserve a food's existing colour.	
Emulsifiers	Allow water and oils to remain mixed together.	Lecithin, alginic acid, carageenan
Flavours	Give food a particular taste or smell.	
Flavour Enhancers	Enhance a food's existing flavours.	Monosodium glutamate (E621)
Flour Treatment Agents	Added to flour to improve its colour or its use in baking.	Ammonium carbonate
Humectants	Prevent foods from drying out.	Sorbitol, mannitol, sodium hydrogen malate
Tracer Gas	Allow for package integrity testing to prevent foods from being exposed to atmosphere, thus guaranteeing shelf life.	
Preservatives	Prevent or inhibit spoilage of food due to fungi, bacteria and other micro-organisms.	Sorbic acid, benzoic acid, sodium benzoate
Stabilizers	Give foods a firmer texture.	Pectin, carageenan
Sweeteners	Sweet flavouring.	Aspartame, saccharin; see page 119
Thickeners	Increase viscosity without substantially modifying its other properties.	Alginic acid, sodium alginate

Stimulants And Anti-Nutrients (25)

On the menu we have:

25 Stimulants And Anti-Nutrients
- Alcohol
  - * Decrease
  - * {Increase} - **unlikely**
- Caffeine
  - * Decrease
  - * {Increase} - **unlikely**
- Tea
  - * Decrease
  - * {Increase} - **unlikely**
- Coffee
  - * Decrease
  - * {Increase} - **unlikely**
- Sugar
  - * Decrease
  - * {Increase} - **unlikely**
- Artificial Sweeteners
  - * Decrease
  - * {Increase} - **unlikely**

Alcohol And Health Problems
Alcohol compromises health in a lot of different ways:

- Alcoholic drinks are empty calories, that is, calories without any nutrients.

- Excess alcohol intake has been linked to mouth, throat, liver, breast, womb and colon cancer.

- Alcohol interferes with our ability to make sound judgements.

- Alcohol is involved in 15% of deaths from road traffic accidents. When people have drunk alcohol, they are usually more confident that they are 'a good driver', but their concentration is worse and their reaction times are slower. If you drive at two times the UK legal limit for alcohol, you are 50 times more likely to be involved in a fatal car crash.

- Severe problems for foetus if mother drinks excess alcohol. Research shows that alcohol (even 3-6 units a week) affects the functioning of the brain of the foetus. (Alcohol Education and Research Council)

- Persistent excess alcohol consumption causes testosterone to drop and damages sperm.

- Alcohol encourages lead absorption and interferes with the absorption of other minerals and some vitamins.

- People who drink heavily tend to have lower levels of some vitamins (A, all the B's and C) and minerals (magnesium and zinc) and essential fatty acids.

- Alcohol stimulates the appetite and increases the flow of gastric juices, so you feel hungrier than you really are. This has implications for people wanting to lose weight.

- Men who drink alcohol appear to have a small increased risk for developing atrial fibrillation, or atrial flutter -- a type of irregular heartbeat.

Current medical advice is that men should restrict their intake to 3-4 units per day, and women should restrict their intake to 2-3 units per day

1 unit of alcohol equals: ½ pint of ordinary beer or small glass of sherry or a glass of wine or a single measure of spirits.

Alcohol And Health Benefits
There has been a lot in the press in the last few years about the health benefits of alcohol. Alcohol consumed in moderation is thought to be beneficial in reducing the risk of coronary heart disease. In 1997, the World Health Organisation concluded that the reduced risk from coronary heart disease was found at the level of one drink consumed every second day.

Caffeine
Caffeine is a stimulant that is in coffee, tea, cola, 'energy drinks' and chocolate. The UK Food Standards Agency urges pregnant women to consume less than 300 mg of caffeine per day.

- 1 mug of instant coffee contains approximately 100mg

- 1 cup of brewed coffee 100mg

- 1 cup of espresso approximately 40 mg

- I cup of decaffeinated coffee approximately 3 mg

- 1 cup of tea is approximately 40 - 50mg

- 1 can of cola is 18-38 mg

- 1 can of 'energy' drink up to 80mg

- 50g bar of plain chocolate up to 50mg

- 50g bar of milk chocolate about 25 mg

(Source: Food Standard Agency and *Nutrition For Life* by Hark and Deen)

Caffeine acts as a diuretic. It is often said that because of this drinking tea and coffee leads to fluid depletion, rather than a fluid increase. Scientific research suggests that this is not true, and that consuming caffeine beverages does increase the amount of fluid in the body. There are other health reasons why it may be wise to reduce the intake of caffeine.

Reducing caffeine rather than reducing coffee or tea will come up on the menu if it is the total amount of caffeine that is important.

Tea
Antioxidants found in tea appear to have a protective effect against cell damage, having a role in preventing heart attacks and possibly cancer. But antioxidants are even more abundant in fruit and vegetables (see page 99).

Tea contains relatively high quantities of manganese. Some people who drink a lot of tea may be doing so in order to provide their bodies with manganese.

The tannins in tea also affects absorption of some minerals.

The UK Food Standards Agency says tea is not a suitable drink for children.

Coffee
Coffee contains central nervous system stimulants and affects mineral absorption.

The UK Food Standards Agency advice is for pregnant women to limit coffee drinking. They also say it is not a suitable drink for children.

Some research has shown that drinking coffee can reduce the risk of type 2 diabetes, Parkinson's disease, colon cancer and gallstones.

Sugar

The health concerns of sugar include:

- Sugar provides only energy and no other nutrients, so an excess intake of sugary foods can reduce the intake of more nutrient-dense foods or else lead to obesity.

- When sugar is broken down for energy, organic acids are produced. This means the body becomes more acid (see page 107).

- Sugar produces a rapid increase in blood sugar levels followed by a sudden decrease in blood sugar levels (see page 200). This encourages the person to eat more foods and drinks that are high in sugar.

Artificial Sweeteners

There have been health concerns about the effect of these chemical sweeteners. There is no unequivocal evidence either way.

Critics also argue that artificial sweeteners, such as aspartame and saccharin, can lead to an increase in the craving for sweet foods, because the sweet taste in the mouth signals to the body that it should prepare for something sweet. When the sweetener does not fulfil this, the body can continue to crave sweet foods.

Allergy (26)

On the menu we have:

26 Allergy
- ➤ Food category (page 17 and Appendix B1 to B3)
  - ＊ Energy work (outside the scope of this book)
  - ＊ Avoid
- ➤ Specific food (page 17)
  - ＊ As above
- ➤ Drink
  - ＊ As above
- ➤ Nutritional supplements
  - ＊ As above
- ➤ Incidentals
  - ＊ As above

What Substances Can Cause A Reaction?

The short answer to this is anything and everything. Contrary to popular belief, it is not just wheat and dairy products and 'junk foods' that cause problems. Some people believe that it is not possible to react to organic products, but many people with hay fever, asthma and allergic rhinitis are reacting to organic grasses and moulds. There is nothing that is safe for everyone. People can be allergic literally to anything, including organic and 'healthy' food. One of my sons was allergic to carrots, including organic carrots – they made him hyperactive. Interestingly he was fine on many of the foods and food additives commonly linked to hyperactivity. One of my clients suffered with migraines, and testing showed she reacted to decaffeinated coffee but not to regular coffee. Presumably it was one of the chemicals used in most decaffeination processes.

Because this is a book on nutritional testing, this allergy section has focussed on nutrition and dietary allergens, but it is also possible for your clients to react to things they inhale or touch. For a more comprehensive analysis of allergens, read my book *Allergy A To Z*.

Do remember that not all allergens are necessarily from the same category. For example you could have a client who is allergic to dairy products (a group), bananas (an individual food), and her washing up liquid (from the incidentals list.)

Which Food Is It?

Before following the systematic questioning plan set out on page 17 onwards, it is better to ask the client what their favourite food is. People are often allergic to foods that they particularly like. Allergies are often addictive, so that people crave the food they react to. It is thought that this is because allergy reactions in the body stimulate endorphin production, and the person gets to like the 'high' that goes with that. Questioning might look like this:

> *Are we looking at allergies next?* Yes
> *Are we looking for foods?* Yes
> *Are we looking for just one food?* Yes
> Is it one of Sam's favourite foods? Yes
> [Ask Sam what his favourite foods are. He says he really likes steak and mushrooms.]
> *Is it either of these?* No
> *Is it something he has at the same time when he eats steak and mushrooms?* No [e.g. could be something in the sauce he always has at the same time.]
> [Ask Sam to name more foods he likes. Also explain that you are using the term 'foods' to cover food and drink. Sam says he really enjoys his glass of orange juice in the morning, likes beer, and is keen on crackers and cheese.]
> *OK, so has Sam named the food we are looking for?* Yes
> [Etc.]

Nutritional Supplement Allergy

Clients can be allergic to their nutritional supplements. It may be the active nutrient (e.g. vitamin B1 or iodine) or one of the excipients (see page 136).

If your client is allergic to a nutrient it may mean that they excrete or store the nutrient inappropriately. In this case, even if there is enough of the nutrient in the diet, the client may be exhibiting deficiency symptoms. Read my book *Energy Mismatch* for a more detailed discussion of this.

Incidentals Allergy

Over the years I have tested thousands of people for allergies, and though most cases have been straight forward, occasionally things got more complicated. Out of this I came up with the category 'incidentals'. This category covers things people do not mean to consume, such as dishwasher chemicals, cutlery, crockery, phthalates (see page 55) migrating from plastic containers into food, etc.

Dishwasher and washing up liquid chemicals do remain on the clean crockery and cutlery and can be a problem for some people. Occasionally clients react to the cutlery itself (often the nickel in stainless steel) or a glaze on the pottery. These are more difficult to comprehend, as it is difficult to see how the metal and glaze, which are relatively inert, end up inside a client's body. But it is my experience that when I correct these problems, it can make a big difference to a client's health.

Once The Allergy Has Been Found

Once the allergy has been found there are several possibilities about what can be done next, depending on your skills. Possibilities include:

- Avoidance: avoiding allergens can work for a while but people often gradually slip back into consuming the substance again. If people do avoid allergens, they often become even more sensitive to the substance if they accidentally ingest it. See page 19 for information on the problems of replacement.

- Energy mismatch procedure: this is explained in my book *Energy Mismatch*, which gives a detailed acupuncture meridian tapping technique for correcting allergies. This procedure comes from Health Kinesiology.

- Other specific allergy correcting techniques: you may know a specific procedure that can correct allergies.

- Indirect correcting allergies: allergies can sometimes be fixed indirectly by focussing on psychological problems or nutritional or structural support, etc.

- Homeopathic or radionically prepared drops or tablets: these are taken by the client usually over several days or several weeks according to a prescribed regime.

Tolerance (27)

On the menu we have:

27 Tolerance
- ➤ Food category (page 17 and Appendix B1 to B3)
  - * Energy work (outside the scope of this book)
  - * Avoid
- ➤ Specific food
  - * As above
- ➤ Drink
  - * As above
- ➤ Nutritional supplements
  - * As above
- ➤ Incidentals
  - * As above

What is the Difference Between Allergy And Tolerance?

If a client has an allergy, this means that they will be sensitive to even the smallest quantity. They may not be consciously aware of a problem, but somewhere within their system the substance has caused a disturbance.

Tolerance problems occur only when the client exceeds their tolerance level for the substance. It is probable that we all have tolerance levels for everything, but if the tolerance level is for twenty oranges a day then in practical terms this will not matter. However, if the tolerance level is for one small orange, whenever a large orange is eaten problems will be experienced. Sometimes tolerance levels are so low that in practical terms the effect is no different from that of an allergy. However, it is different in terms of what is happening in the energy system, and so has to be tested for separately and corrected differently.

As with allergy, tolerance can be to a food, or drink, a nutritional supplement or to something incidental. (Looked at from a wider perspective it can also be to something inhaled or through contact.)

Testing For Tolerance Levels

There are two steps:

- Identifying the substance: done in the same was as for allergies (see page 120).
- Identifying the maximum that is allowed.

The maximum that is tolerated will vary. Tolerance levels are not set rigidly. They will vary with stress. So, if a client is short of sleep, their tolerance will be lower. If they have an infection, had an argument or not taking good care of themselves, their tolerance levels will decrease. This makes testing difficult. In general the easiest way to test is to test for the tolerance given the 'normal' amount of stress in the client's life.

For example, having identified that the client has a tolerance problem with oranges, the maximum quantity needs to be established. First ask the client how they would like you to measure the oranges. (See also page 38). With foods like oranges there can be a problem because oranges may be eaten in several different formats – oranges as a whole fruit, as fruit juice and (if your client is English) marmalade. If the client never eats marmalade, this can be excluded from the calculations, so you need to ask the client what forms the client eats the item in. It is often necessary to prompt them with where the substance can be found. It is surprising how ignorant people can be. I have had clients, for example, who think that wheat is only found in bread and need to be told/reminded that it is also in pasta, breakfast cereals, etc. My book *Allergy A To Z* can help with this. So, for the sake of this exercise we will look at a client that eats oranges in all three forms. The easiest way is to take the main source and find the amount for this and then ask about the combinations. It is usually not necessary to do every possible permutation, but give the client a feel of the possibilities. So testing might look like this:

> *Looking at oranges on their own and with an 'average' amount of stress in Ann's life, what is Ann's maximum tolerance for oranges per day - More than 2?* No
> *More than 1?* Yes
> *So, it is 2 oranges?* Yes
> *If Ann eats 1 orange a day, how much marmalade can she eat - more than 2 slices of toast and marmalade?* Yes
> [This is a rather unconventional measure of marmalade, but the client finds it the most practical rather than measuring in teaspoonfuls or by weight; note though that this only works if the client uses the same size slice of bread all the time.]
> *More than 3 slices of toast and marmalade?* No
> *So, it's 3 slices of toast?* No
> *So it's two and a half slices of toast and marmalade is that correct?* Yes
> So Ann can eat one orange and have two and a half slices of toast and marmalade a day without any problem – is that correct? Yes
> [Work out other combinations.]
> *Would it be appropriate to work out levels for Ann when she's working extra long hours?* Yes

[You know that this client has a very demanding job and goes through periods several times a year when she works very long hours. For another client the question might be about times when she's arguing with her boyfriend, or travelling away from home, etc.]
So, looking at oranges on their own, when Ann works long hours, is Ann's tolerance for oranges less than 2? Yes
Less than 1? No
[Etc.]

The second part of the questioning about what happens when clients are particularly stressed can act as a real lever to help them make changes in their lives. You could also test, as well or instead, for what consumption would be when there is very little stress.

It is important at the end of questioning on tolerance to check that the clients know what they need to do and also that they understand that the amounts are maximum not optimum.

Vital Energy (28)

On the menu we have:

28 Vital Energy
- ➤ Avoid /Decrease
  - ∗ Food
  - ∗ Drink
  - ∗ Nutritional supplements
  - ∗ Incidentals
- ➤ Start/Increase
  - ∗ Food
  - ∗ Drink
  - ∗ Nutritional supplements
  - ∗ Incidentals

What Is Vital Energy?

Vital energy is the life force, also called Chi or prana. Our vital energy is our underlying reserve of life energy. Shocks, accidents and surgery can suddenly and massively reduce our vital energy, but our underlying vital energy levels tend to remain the same over long periods of time. Temporary changes can be a result of taking in a substance that has a low vital energy for us.

In an ideal world you would only eat, drink and take in substances that enhance your vital energy. If you are allergic to something or exceeding your tolerance level for it, it will not enhance your vital energy. But substances can lower your vital energy for other reasons too. It depends on the vital energy of the substance in relation to your own vital energy. So, for example, vegetables that have been cooked for a long time would probably not enhance most people's vital energy. But if you were starving or did not normally eat any fruit and vegetables, such a food could in these circumstances enhance your vital energy.

Testing For Vital Energy

The procedure in many ways is similar as that for tolerance except now there are two possibilities:

- ▪ Identifying substances that have a negative effect on the client's vital energy.
- ▪ Identifying substances that have a positive effect on the client's vital energy.

The substance could be a whole category or an individual substance. I usually find out first whether I am testing for negative or positive effects, as certain foods etc. might then suggest themselves. If you are testing for negative vital energy, you will be looking for the maximum that can be consumed without a detrimental effect. For the positive effect you are usually looking for optimum amount, although occasionally you may want to find the minimum amount that will have a beneficial effect. Testing might look like this:

So, is Vital Energy next? Yes
Are we looking at positive effect? Yes
Is this a single food? Yes
[Etc.]

Specific Dietary Programmes (29)

On the menu we have:

29 Specific Dietary Programme
- ➤ Vegetarian
- ➤ Vegan
- ➤ Macrobiotic
- ➤ Blood Group Diet
- ➤ Atkins Diet *(page 197)*
- ➤ Other

Client Already Following A Specific Diet

Sometimes the client is already following a particular dietary regime, and this needs to be modified in some way. This could come up here, or directly in some other way. So, for example, if your client was following a macrobiotic diet, you could get to 'reduce (or increase) the amount of seaweed you eat' in several different ways:

- It could come up via this part of the nutritional testing menu as a modification on the standard diet.

- It could come up via the intolerance section of the menu. (See page 123.)

- It could come up via the vital energy section of the menu. (See page 126.)

Starting A Special Diet

If testing shows that the client should follow a specific diet, test whether it is the dietary regime in their totality, or whether it needs to be modified.

Vegetarians

Some people say they are vegetarian even though they eat fish and chicken, so it is important to establish exactly what the person means when they say that they are a vegetarian.

In general vegetarians:

- Do not eat meat, fish, poultry but will eat dairy products and eggs
- Some will not eat cheese made with animal rennet
- Some will not use supplements and medicines in gelatine-based capsules
- Some will not eat battery eggs

Vegetarians need to make sure their intakes of zinc and iron are sufficient either by eating acceptable foods rich in these or by taking supplements.

Vegans

Vegans do not eat meat, fish, poultry, dairy products, eggs. Some will also not eat honey.

Vegans need to eat mixtures of plant proteins to give an appropriate amino acid combination; e.g.

- Cereals + pulses.
- Nuts/seeds + pulses.
- Cereals + nuts/seeds.
- Vegetables + pulses.

Recent research now suggests that it is not necessary for the combination to be consumed at the same meal as was once thought. (See page 73 for more on amino acids.)

Vegans also need to make sure their intake of zinc, calcium, iron and B12 are sufficient either by eating acceptable foods rich in these or by taking supplements.

Macrobiotic Diet

This is promoted as a therapeutic diet. The macrobiotic diet attempts to balance yin (e.g. root vegetables) and yang (e.g. fruit) foods. In this system rice is thought to be the perfectly balanced food, so people following a macrobiotic diet will sometimes eat only brown rice for a while. More generally:

- Organically grown food is eaten wherever possible.
- Vegetables are sliced and cooked in a special manner.
- Raw food is felt to be too indigestible.
- Extensive use is made of sea vegetables, pulses and fermented rice and soya products.
- Fruit is kept to less than 5% of diet.

- Bread and pasta intake is limited.

- Dairy foods, eggs, members of the nightshade family (e.g. potatoes, tomatoes, peppers), baked goods, sugar, refined foods and high fat foods are usually avoided.

Blood Type Diet

Promoted as a therapeutic diet. The main popular book on this is *Eat Right For Your Type* by Peter J D'Adamo, N.D. The theory is that the different blood groups have developed at different times in mankind's history:

Type 0	40,000 years ago
Type A	20,000 years ago
Type B	10,000 years ago
Type AB	1,000 years ago

It is argued that because they developed at different times, the ideal diet for people with that blood type is akin to what was available at the time of its emergence:

- Type O The Hunter: good digestive tract and an over-active immune system. This type should eat mostly meat, poultry and seafood, but avoid dairy products and cereal products.
- Type A The Cultivator: sensitive digestive tract and tolerant immune system. Avoid meat, eat poultry, avoid dairy products, no wheat but other breads are generally OK.
- Type B The Nomad: strong immune system and tolerant digestive system. Eat dairy foods. Avoid beef, wheat and all shell fish.
- Type AB The Enigma: sensitive digestive tract. Over tolerant immune system. Eat most meat (but not beef or chicken), wheat and some dairy.

Peter D'Adamo does not recommend taking supplements:

> "a supplement is considered an avoid because it is bountiful in a well rounded, fresh food based diet for your blood type"

and

> "the vast majority of those with positive outcomes were not using supplements, while those taking supplements were not seeing similar results"

Both quotations are taken from his web site (www.dadamo.com).

Criticisms Of This Approach:

- It is likely that some of the beneficial results reported by people on these diets are because they are avoiding one or more allergens rather than the whole diet making the difference.

- When asked about people who are allergic/intolerant to beneficial foods for their blood type, Peter D'Adamo says that these occur because of drugs, surgery or disease. This cannot be proved and is a convenient explanation for all the people who do not fit the theory.

- The problems with wheat (an avoid for virtually all blood types) may be because wheat has been selectively bred to increase its protein content and not because there is a problem with wheat as such.

- A lot of the information in the book is presented as scientific fact, but some scientists have said there is not good scientific evidence for it, e.g. the effect of lectins on muscle tissues.

- His assertions about lectins and blood clumping are based on work with blood on slides. What happens in the body is not necessarily the same. Some enzymes (such as intestinal transglutaminase) can repair any damage caused by lectins. If red blood cells do agglutinate (stick together/clump) as a result of lectins in some foods, this is potentially life-threatening and "pathologists and other medical scientists would be familiar with a syndrome of organ failure due to lectin-induced micro-infarctions (cell death)." Michael Klaper, M.D. (www.veg.on.ca/lifelines/janfeb/blood.htm)

- Part of the justification for saying O types should eat meat is that they have high stomach acid. Not all O types do have high stomach acid.

- Some information is wrong, e.g. that the body produces iodine.

- Some of his information on the environment and food when the blood types emerged may be wrong. Historical evidence suggests that all blood types developed before the introduction of agriculture and all have lived through the hunter-gatherer period and so have been subjected to the same influences.

Testing For A Specific Diet

If this comes up in testing, you need to establish first which diet is to be followed, and then check if it needs to be modified in some way. The Food Combining section on page 103 shows how this might be done.

Supplements (30)

On the menu we have:

30 Supplements
- ➢ Check existing supplements
  - * Beneficial and optimal
  - * Beneficial but not optimal
  - * Beneficial but something about it needs to be changed
  - * Harmful
  - * Neither beneficial or harmful
- ➢ New Supplements
  - * Specific Manufacturer
  - * Vitamins (page 90 and Appendix A1)
  - * Minerals (page 94 and Appendix A2)
  - * Amino Acid (page 73)
  - * Oils (page 79)
  - * Antioxidants (page 99)
  - * Prebiotics And Probiotics (page 101)
- ➢ Other

Why Take Supplements?

Many authorities argue that providing you eat 'a balanced diet' you do not need to take supplements, but there is mounting evidence that many people can benefit from taking supplements:

- Allergies and tolerance problems can lead to an inadequate diet.

- Unwillingness to eat a healthy diet will lead to nutritional deficiencies.

- Relying on snacks and take-aways because "busy".

- Dieting unwisely.

- Over cooking food, either initially or reheating.

- Illness can affect absorption, e.g. coeliac disease alters lining of small intestine so less efficient uptake of nutrients.

- Sub-clinical problems of the digestive system can lead to problems of absorption.

- Some people, because of biochemical individuality, have problems absorbing a particular nutrient even without a "clinical disease".

- Healing processes require more nutrients for detoxifying and repair.

- Puberty and pregnancy increase the need for nutrients.

- Inappropriate habits: e.g. excess coffee interferes with B vitamin absorption; smokers need more vitamin C.

- Exercise increases the need for nutrients, but this is not a reason not to exercise.

- Taking drugs can affect the need for nutrients. (See page 190)

- Pollution has led to an increase in the need for antioxidants in the diet. (See page 99)

- Most soil is now depleted of trace minerals, because food is grown repeatedly in the same place and only some nutrients are replaced.

Accuracy

The most accurate way of testing supplements is to have a supplement there while you ask the question. Many manufacturers now provide testing kits of their supplements, and these allow you to have access to a wide range of supplements without incurring a great deal of expense. Some branches of kinesiology teach that the supplement should be put on the client's body while the testing takes place. I generally like to have it in my hand or close by while testing verbal questions.

If the client brings an unfamiliar supplement in for testing, I normally read what it says on the label, take a capsule out, look at it and smell it before starting the questioning.

There are occasions when you want to do some questioning but do not have a supplement available. In general you will get more accurate answers if you and/or the client have experience of the supplement. Testing off lists when neither you nor the client has any experience of the supplement is likely to be the least accurate.

What Are You Testing For?

You need to be clear in your mind before you start supplement testing what standard you are testing to:

- Supplements needed to avoid gross deficiency signs.

- Supplements to maintain or improve general health and well-being.

- Supplements for a particular problem (e.g. acne, osteoarthritis).

Two Different Situations

There are two main possibilities:

- The person may already be taking supplements and you want to check if everything is correct.

- The person may not be taking any supplements at all.

The procedure I recommend is slightly different depending on which of these situations you have.

Client Already Taking Supplements

First look at the existing supplements that are being taken. There are five basic possibilities for each supplement:

- It is beneficial and optimal.

- It is beneficial but not the best one to take (e.g. client does need a multi-vitamin supplement but not the one they are currently taking).

- It is beneficial, and the best source, but something about it needs to be changed (dose, time taken, avoid / have at same time, etc.).

- It is harmful.

- It is having no effect.

For each supplement ask which of these categories applies. If the second option, you need to find an alternative either from the same manufacturer or from an alternative manufacturer. If the third option, work out what needs changing, e.g.

> *Is this vitamin C supplement beneficial and optimal?* No
> *Beneficial but not best source?* No
> *Beneficial but something needs to be changed?* Yes
> *Is the dose correct?* Yes
> *Is the time that it's taken correct?* No [Client takes in the morning on an empty stomach.]
> *Should the vitamin C supplement be taken with food?* Yes
> *Do we need to know anything else about the vitamin C supplement?* Yes
> *At a particular meal?* Yes
> Breakfast? Yes
> *So the vitamin C supplement should be taken with breakfast? Is that correct?* Yes
> *Anything else we need to know about the vitamin C supplement?* No

When you have checked each supplement the client is currently taking, ask if any others need to be added, and if so follow the same procedure as for clients who are not taking anything to find the additional supplements.

Client Not Taking Any Supplements At The Moment

Check first of all that the client needs to take supplements.
It is possible to work out the supplements in two different ways:

- Finding the type of nutrient first e.g. 500 mg of vitamin C and then finding a supplement that matches this.

- Finding the supplement that is best.

In general the second approach is the easiest, e.g.

> *Do I have a sample of this supplement here?* Yes
> *Is it one of brand X?* No
> *Is it one of brand Y?* Yes
> [Etc.]

If it is a supplement that you do not have there, you can ask if it is one that you know about or the client knows about.

Once you have found the supplement, you need to check what the dose is and how it should be taken. Normally you first look at the standard does that is recommended by the manufacturer, and ask:

> *Do you take the supplement as detailed on the packet?* Yes

You then ask:

> *Is there anything else we need to know about this supplement?*

It could be that there is some additional instruction that is necessary. For example, the manufacturer's instruction might say that the standard dose is one tablet a day with food, but the full instruction for the client could be one tablet a day with food, and the client should also eat some vitamin C rich food at the same time to enhance absorption.

If the client does not take the supplement as indicated on the packet, you would need to work out all the details of dose and timing, e.g.

> *Do you take at least two tablets a day?* Yes
> *More than two?* No
> *Are both tablets taken at the same time?* No
> *Is one or both taken with meals?* Yes
> [Etc.]

Issues Of Cost

Supplements cost money, and some clients may not feel they can afford to pay for a full programme of supplements, but this has to be their decision not the therapists. It is possible to ask the question:

If money were no object, what is the ideal supplement programme?

Once you have worked this out, you can then discuss with the client what to do. An alternative and probably better approach practically is to talk to a client of limited means about how much they feel able to spend on supplements and then test to this, e.g.

Vera wants to spend a maximum of £X per month on supplements, so what are the best ones for her to take given this constraint?

Cheap Supplements

There are many cheap supplements around and undoubtedly some of them are very good value, but cheap supplements are not always the best:

- Oils are often extracted with hexane (a solvent) that can leave traces in the supplement.

- Oils may be extracted using heat that can damage the integrity of the oil.

- Herbal extracts may contain the non-active part of the plant as this is often cheaper.

Other Ingredients In Supplements

Inactive ingredients are used in the making of many tablets and capsules. These excipients are part of the manufacturing process to ensure that the supplement is accurately made and consistent in form and may also aid digestion and absorption in some way.

Possible excipients include:

- Diluents: dilute the nutrient so that it can be accurately dispersed in the tablets or capsules. Diluents include microcrystalline cellulose, dicalcium phosphate, soya oil.

- Coatings: these are used to mask the taste of the nutrients and make them easier to swallow. Coatings include shellac (from a beetle), hydroxypropylmethyl cellulose, natural colourants (such as chlorophyll and iron oxide) and magnesium silicate.

- Plasticisers: used in soft-gel capsules to impart suppleness. Glycerin is a plasticiser.

- Disintegrants: produce a "matrix" throughout the tablet that can be acted upon by fluids in the digestive system. There are European standards for disintegration (15 minutes for uncoated tablets; 30 minutes for coated tablets). Disintegrants include modified cellulose and soya fibre.

- Lubricants/flow aids: ensures that powders flow through machinery during manufacture. Lubricants include magnesium stearate, stearic acid, hydrogenated vegetable oil and silica in the form of silicon dioxide.

(The information on excipients is supplied by Lamberts Healthcare Ltd)

Testing For Supplements

Testing for supplements may seem like a very straight-forward process, because it is easy not to be precise in the questions you ask. Here are a number of important considerations:

- What are we testing for? Optimum dose, adequate dose, minimum dose, dose in relation to a particular problem. Depending on the circumstances different options may be more or less appropriate.

- What make and form of the supplement? E.g. the client might absorb zinc citrate better than zinc amino acid chelate.

- Is the client allergic to this supplement? If not, the problem may be with the nutrient itself and/or one of the other ingredients. (See pages 120 and 136.)

- Can the person tolerate the dose proposed? It may be the nutrient itself and/or one of the other ingredients. (See pages 123 and 136.)

- Will this particular version of the supplement enhance the client's life force? (See page 126.)

- Are any other nutrients necessary at the same time? Would any other nutrient help absorption? e.g. zinc is necessary for absorption of evening primrose oil; vitamin C enhances iron absorption.

- Timing? Some nutritional supplements need to be taken with food, while others should be taken away from food. Some need to be taken early in the day and some at bedtime. Appendix A1 and A2 give some information on what is usual, but testing can determine what is optimum for the person.

- With or without anything else. E.g. tea interferes with absorption of zinc so should not be drunk close to the time when a zinc supplement is taken.

- Chewed/ swallowed? E.g. most calcium supplements are best swallowed; most herbs are best tasted in the mouth before being swallowed.

- How long should the supplement be taken for? It is possible that the dose will need to be increased/ decreased at a future date.

- Will the client actually take the supplements? If a lot of supplements are needed, but the client cannot afford to buy them, then need to ask about priority of supplements. Some people will not take supplements containing animal products such as gelatine. Some people have difficulty swallowing large tablets/ capsules.

- Circumstances may change, so it is necessary to check that the supplement schedule is still correct for that person.

References: Books

Allergy A to Z, Jane Thurnell-Read, Life-Work Potential, 2005, ISBN 978-0954243920

The Allergy Survival Guide, Jane Houlton, Leopard Books, 1995, ISBN 978-0752900230

Biochemistry & Molecular Biology, W.H & D.C. Elliott, OUP, 2001, ISBN 978-0198700456

The Complete Guide To Food Allergy & Intolerance Prof. Jonathan Brostoff and Linda Gamlin, Quality Health Books, 2008, ISBN 978-1906680008

The Complete Illustrated Guide To Nutritional Healing, Denise Mortimore, Element Books, 1998, ISBN 978-0760711675

Eating Well For Optimum Health Dr Andrew Weil, Sphere 2008, ISBN 978-0751540826

E For Additives, Maurice Hanssen with Jill Marsden, 1987, Thorsons, ISBN 978-0722515624

The Encyclopedia of Natural Medicine, Michael T. Murray and Joseph E. Pizzorno, Prima Publishing, 1999, ISBN978-0761511571

The Encyclopedia Of Nutritional Supplements, Michael T Murray, Prima Publishing, 1996, ISBN 978-0761504108

Energy Mismatch, Jane Thurnell-Read, Life-Work Potential, 2004, ISBN 978-0954243937

Food Combining for Health, Doris Grant and Jean Joice, Thorsons, 1991, ISBN 978-0722525067

The New Glucose Revolution Dr Anthony Leeds and Jennie Brand Miller, Mobius, ISBN 978-0340827024

Manual of Nutrition, Food Standards Agency, Stationery Office Books, 2008, ISBN 978-0112431169

Nutrient Content of Food Portions, Jill Davies and John Dickerson, Royal Society of Chemistry, 1991. ISBN 978-0851864266

Nutrition For Life, Lisa Hark and Dr Darwin Deen, Dorling Kindersley, 2005, ISBN 978-1405303064

The Nutritional Health Bible, Linda Lazarides, Thorsons, 1997, ISBN 978-0722534243

Nutrition Matters for Practice Nurses, Anthony Leeds et al, John Libbey & Co. Ltd, 1990, ISBN 978-0861962822

Nutrition in Primary Care, Briony Thomas, Wiley Blackwell, 1996 ISBN 978-0632039814

The Optimum Nutrition Bible, Patrick Holford, Piatkus, 2004, ISBN 978-0749925529

The Practitioner's Guide To Supplements, Lamberts Healthcare Ltd.

Staying Healthy with Nutrition, Dr Elson Haas, Celestial Arts, 2006, ISBN 978-1587611797

Thorsons Complete Guide To Vitamins & Minerals Leonard Mervyn, Thorsons, 2000, ISBN 978-0722539774

Verbal Questioning Skills For Kinesiologists, Jane Thurnell-Read, Life-Work Potential, 2004, ISBN 978-0954243913

WCRF Guide to Vitamins, World Cancer Research Fund (leaflet)

The WDDTY Good Supplement Guide, 2003 What Doctors Don't Tell You Ltd.

You Are What You Eat Kirsten Hartvig and Dr Nic Rowley, Piatkus, 2003, 978-0749924027

References: Web Sites

British Dietetics Association
www.bda.uk.com

Linus Pauling Institute, Oregon State University, USA
http://lpi.oregonstate.edu/

Medline Plus
www.nlm.nih.gov/medlineplus

National Institutes Of Health, Office Of Dietary Supplements
http://dietary-supplements.info.nih.gov/

UK Foods Standard Agency
http://www.food.gov.uk

Wikipedia
www.wikipedia.org

Appendix A1: Vitamins

Vitamin A/ Retinol

Please note that this information is indicative rather than comprehensive, serving as a reminder rather than a full explanation of the nature and role of this vitamin.

Fat-Soluble

Good Sources
Liver, eggs, milk & dairy products, fish liver oil, enriched margarine, carrots, parsley, spinach, broccoli.

Functions
Growth and repair of body tissues; bone and tooth formation; vision in dim light; keeps mucus membranes healthy; helps immune system; protection from some cancers; works as an antioxidant (see page 99).

Possible Deficiency Effects
Reduced night vision; dry eyes; loss of vision due to gradual damage of cornea; poor wound healing; eczema; dermatitis; scaly dry flaky skin; pale skin; reduced resistance to infection due to loss of integrity of skin and mucus membranes; follicular hyperkeratosis; reduced sense of taste.

Possible Toxic Effects
Headaches; drowsiness; skin changes; anorexia; weight loss; muscle pain; chronic liver disease; itchy and flaky skin; loss of body hair; brittle nails; blurred vision; increased risk of birth defects in pregnant women.

Intake
Upper safe limit for long-term use: 2300 mcg per day

Remarks
Vitamin A can be made in the body from the provitamin carotene.
Absorption hindered by lack of bile.

Supplements
Take with fatty food.
Absorption helped by zinc, vitamins E & C.
Supplements above 2000 i.u. should be avoided by pregnant women

Beta-Carotene

Please note that this information is indicative rather than comprehensive, serving as a reminder rather than a full explanation of the nature and role of this vitamin.

Fat-Soluble

Good Sources
Yellow and green fruit & vegetables.

Functions
Free-radical scavenger; antioxidant properties; protection against some cancers

Possible Deficiency Effects
Same as vitamin A

Possible Toxic Effects
Same as vitamin A

Remarks
Converted to Vitamin A in the body; some research has suggested beta-carotene increases the risk of cancers in smokers.

Vitamin B1/ Thiamin

Please note that this information is indicative rather than comprehensive, serving as a reminder rather than a full explanation of the nature and role of this vitamin.

Water- Soluble

Good Sources
Wheat germ, yeast, liver, whole grains, brazil nuts, peanuts, soya flour, oatmeal, lentils, fish, poultry, beans, pork.

Functions
Carbohydrate metabolism; appetite maintenance; nerve function; growth and muscle tone; important for heart.

Possible Deficiency Effects
Tiredness; depression; irritability; inability to concentrate; poor memory; sore and aching muscles; gastrointestinal disturbances; numbness and tingling in hands and feet; swollen legs (fluid retention); reduced pain tolerance; disturbed sleep; weight loss; poor appetite; rapid heart beat; congestive heart failure; poor growth in children.

Intake
Upper safe limit for long-term use: 100 mg per day.
UK RDA: 1 mg for men and 0.8 mg for women.

Supplements
All the B vitamins work together, so often best taken as a B complex formulation.
Take early in day.
Absorption helped by other B vitamins and manganese.
Absorption hindered by alcohol, stress and antibiotics.
Seek medical advice first if taking the drug L-Dopa.
Diabetics should not take doses over 75mg daily without consulting their doctor

Vitamin B2 / Riboflavin

Please note that this information is indicative rather than comprehensive, serving as a reminder rather than a full explanation of the nature and role of this vitamin.

Water- Soluble

Good Sources
Fortified breakfast cereals, meat, eggs, almonds, blue cheese, mushrooms, green leafy vegetables, offal, nuts.

Functions
Fat, carbohydrate and protein metabolism; formation of antibodies and red blood cells.

Possible Deficiency Effects
Sore tongue and lips; cracks in skin around nose and mouth; sore or bleeding gums; blood shot, itchy, watery eyes; sensitivity to bright lights; burning feet; red and greasy skin but also dryness and flaking; scrotal and vulval dermatitis; pale skin; dull or oily hair; brittle and split fingernails; spoon-shaped (concave) nails.

Intake
Upper safe limit for long-term use: 200 mg per day.
UK RDA: 1.3 mg for men and 1.1 mg for women.

Supplements
All the B vitamins work together, so often best taken as a B complex formulation.
Take early in day.
Absorption helped by other B vitamins.
Absorption hindered by alcohol, stress and antibiotics.
Seek medical advice first if taking the drug L-Dopa.
Large doses may affect blood tests.

Vitamin B3 / Niacin/ Nicotinic Acid / Nicotinamide

Please note that this information is indicative rather than comprehensive, serving as a reminder rather than a full explanation of the nature and role of this vitamin.

Water- Soluble

Good Sources
Meat, poultry, fish, liver, milk products, peanuts, almonds, potatoes, yeast extract, hard cheese, haricot beans.

Functions
Fat, carbohydrate and protein metabolism; health of nerves, skin, tongue and digestive system; blood circulation.

Possible Deficiency Effects
Irritability; lack of energy; weight loss; poor appetite; headaches; poor memory; lack of concentration; emotional instability; redness, scaling & pigmentation of skin in light-exposed areas; scaly dry flaky skin; sore & fissured tongue; cracking at corners of mouth; abdominal pain; diarrhoea.

Possible Toxic Effects
Flushing; peptic ulcers; liver dysfunction; gout; arrhythmia; hyperglycaemia.

Intake
Upper safe limit for long-term use: 150 mg per day.
UK RDA: 17 mg for men and 13 mg for women.

Remarks
Niacin can be synthesised by the body from tryptophan (see page 78).

Supplements
All the B vitamins work together, so often best taken as a B complex formulation.
Take early in day.
Absorption helped by other B vitamins.
Absorption hindered by alcohol, stress and antibiotics.
Seek medical advice first if taking the drug L-Dopa.
Diabetics should not take doses over 75mg daily without consulting their doctor.
Doses over 100 mg may aggravate stomach ulcers, glaucoma and diabetes.

Vitamin B5 / Pantothenic Acid

Please note that this information is indicative rather than comprehensive, serving as a reminder rather than a full explanation of the nature and role of this vitamin.

Water- Soluble

Good Sources
Meat, whole grains, legumes, yeast.

Functions
Converts nutrients into energy; formation of some fats; vitamin utilisation; production of hormones and cholesterol.

Possible Deficiency Effects
Tiredness; headaches; weakness; emotional swings; muscle cramps; nausea.

Supplements
All the B vitamins work together, so often best taken as a B complex formulation.
Take early in day.
Absorption helped by other B vitamins and specifically biotin and folic acid.
Absorption hindered by stress and antibiotics.
Seek medical advice first if taking the drug L-Dopa.

Vitamin B6 / Pyridoxine

Please note that this information is indicative rather than comprehensive, serving as a reminder rather than a full explanation of the nature and role of this vitamin.

Water- Soluble

Good Sources
Fish, poultry, lean meat, whole grain cereals, walnuts, butterbeans, bananas, peanuts.

Functions
Fat, carbohydrate and protein metabolism; formation of antibodies; maintains sodium/ potassium balance; increases the amount of oxygen carried by haemoglobin.

Possible Deficiency Effects
Exacerbates anaemia; irritability; nervousness; depression; insomnia; seborrhoeic dermatitis on face; acne-like rash on forehead; red and greasy skin but also dryness and flaking; sore tongue; prominent taste buds; lack of energy.

Possible Toxic Effects
Impairment of sensory nerve function; diminished tendon reflexes; numbness and loss of sensations in hands and feet; difficulty in walking.

Intake
Upper safe limit for long-term use: 100 mg per day.
UK RDA for men: 1.4 mg and 1.2 mg for women.

Remarks
Increased requirement in women premenstrually and those taking the contraceptive pill.
The more protein in the diet the more vitamin B6 is needed to help the body use the protein.

Supplements
All the B vitamins work together, so often best taken as a B complex formulation.
Take early in day.
Absorption helped by other B vitamins, magnesium and zinc.
Absorption hindered by alcohol, stress and antibiotics.
Seek medical advice first if taking the drug L-Dopa.
Doses over 100 mg may cause peripheral neuritis.

Vitamin B12 / Cyanocobalamin / Cobalamin

Please note that this information is indicative rather than comprehensive, serving as a reminder rather than a full explanation of the nature and role of this vitamin.

Water- Soluble

Good sources
Offal, eggs, milk, oily fish, cheese.

Functions
Works with folic acid (see page 153). Fat, carbohydrate and protein metabolism; maintains health of nervous system; blood cell formation; folate synthesis; DNA synthesis.

Possible Deficiency Effects
Pernicious anaemia; mental confusion; irritability; anxiety; tiredness; pale skin; recurrent mouth ulcers; sore and inflamed tongue; scaly dry flaky skin; poor hair condition; diarrhoea; sore and tender muscles; tingling in ands and feet.

Intake
Upper safe limit for long-term use: 300 mcg per day.
UK RDA: 0.0015 mg.

Remarks
Vitamin B12 has to be combined with intrinsic factor produced in the stomach in order to be absorbed. Pernicious anaemia usually involves lack of intrinsic factor for absorption of B12 (associated with blue eyes and prematurely grey hair).

Supplements
All the B vitamins work together, so often best taken as a B complex formulation.
Take early in day.
Absorption helped by other B vitamins, particularly folic acid, and calcium.
Absorption hindered by alcohol, stress, internal parasites and antibiotics.
Seek medical advice first if taking the drug L-Dopa.
High intakes may mask folic acid deficiency.
High levels of supplementation should be avoided in pregnancy and by under 12's.

Biotin - Classified as both Vitamin H and as a B Vitamin

Please note that this information is indicative rather than comprehensive, serving as a reminder rather than a full explanation of the nature and role of this vitamin.

Water- Soluble

Good Sources
Yeast, offal, eggs, milk, cheese, soya beans, peanuts, walnuts, beans, cauliflower.

Functions
Fat, carbohydrate and protein metabolism; helps utilise B vitamins; involved in production of hormones and cholesterol (see page 87); healthy hair, nails and skin.

Possible Deficiency Effects
Scaly dermatitis; tiredness; weakness; poor appetite; pale skin; poor hair condition; hair loss; sore and aching muscles; severe cradle cap in infants.

Intake
No RDA but 30 to 100 mcg a day appears to be sufficient.

Remarks
Made by the bacteria in the gut (see page 101). Long-term antibiotics can cause biotin deficiency.

Supplements
All the B vitamins work together, so often best taken as a B complex formulation.
Take early in day.
Absorption helped by other B vitamins.
Absorption hindered by stress, raw egg white and antibiotics.
Seek medical advice first if taking the drug L-Dopa.

Choline

Please note that this information is indicative rather than comprehensive, serving as a reminder rather than a full explanation of the nature and role of this vitamin.

Water- Soluble

Good Sources
Widely available in food.

Functions
Part of formation of acetylcholine; emulsifies fats.

Remarks
Can be synthesised from glycine.

Supplements
All the B vitamins work together, so often best taken as a B complex formulation.
Take early in day.
Absorption helped by vitamin B5.
Absorption hindered by alcohol, stress and antibiotics.
Seek medical advice first if taking the drug L-Dopa.

Inositol

Please note that this information is indicative rather than comprehensive, serving as a reminder rather than a full explanation of the nature and role of this vitamin.

Water- Soluble

Good Sources
Widely available in food.

Functions
Emulsifies fats.

Possible Deficiency Effects
Poor hair condition; eczema; benefits diabetics; Supplementation may benefit people suffering from problems such as bulimia, panic disorder, bipolar depression and polycystic ovary syndrome (PCOS).

Remarks
Can be synthesised from glucose; caffeine can produce deficiency of inositol.

Supplements
All the B vitamins work together, so often best taken as a B complex formulation.
Take early in day.
Absorption helped by choline.
Absorption hindered by alcohol, stress and antibiotics.
Seek medical advice first if taking the drug L-Dopa.

Folic Acid / Folate / Folacin

Please note that this information is indicative rather than comprehensive, serving as a reminder rather than a full explanation of the nature and role of this vitamin.

Water- Soluble

Good Sources
Green leafy vegetables, offal, melons, pumpkins, peanuts, butter beans, carrots, egg yolk, apricots, avocado, tomatoes, broccoli, spinach, asparagus.

Functions
Folate works with vitamin B12 (see page 149) to help form red blood cells; necessary for the production of DNA, which controls tissue growth and cell function.

Possible Deficiency Effects
Megaloblastic anaemia; neural tube defects where mother's intake not adequate; poor growth in children; cracks at corners of mouth; scaly dry flaky skin; painful sore tongue; mouth ulcers; depression; lack of energy; poor appetite; diarrhoea.

Possible Toxic Effects
Insomnia, irritability.

Intake
Upper safe limit for long-term use: 400 mcg per day.
UK RDA: 0.2 mg; for pregnant women 0.4 mg.

Remarks
Supplementation can mask B12 deficiency.
Increased requirement in women taking the contraceptive pill.
Increased requirements in the first 12 weeks of pregnancy (see page 187).

Supplements
All the B vitamins work together, so often best taken as a B complex formulation.
Take early in day.
Absorption helped by other B vitamins and vitamin C.
Absorption hindered by alcohol, stress and antibiotics.
Seek medical advice first if taking the drug L-Dopa.
High intakes may mask B12 deficiency.

Vitamin C / Ascorbic Acid

Please note that this information is indicative rather than comprehensive, serving as a reminder rather than a full explanation of the nature and role of this vitamin.

Water- Soluble

Good Sources
Citrus fruit, nectarines, strawberries, melons, vegetables, tomatoes, potatoes. Most other fruits and vegetables contain some vitamin C; fish and milk contain small amounts.

Functions
Helps heal wounds; strengthens blood vessels; collagen maintenance; resistance to infection; required for production of adrenal hormones; helps detoxification and excretion of a wide range of toxic chemicals; aids absorption of iron; works as an antioxidant (see page 99).

Possible Deficiency Effects
Scurvy; poor wound healing; lowered resistance to infection; easy bruising; small red or purple spots on the skin; bleeding gums; fragile capillaries; damage to bone & connective tissue; dry and scaly skin; dandruff; fatigue; shortness of breath on exertion; aching or weak bones; joint pain; depression; delayed teething in babies.

Possible Toxic Effects
Diarrhoea; kidney stones because of increased excretion of water and oxolate; impairment of white cell function; decreased B12 and increased iron absorption.

Intake
Upper safe limit for long-term use: 200 mg per day.
UK RDA: 40 mg.

Remarks
Aspirin, barbiturates, corticosteroids, tetracycline drugs increase excretion.

Supplements
Best taken between meals.
Absorption hindered by heavy metals and inadequate hydrochloric acid in the stomach.
High intake can cause diarrhoea, stomach cramps and flatulence.
High doses of vitamin C as ascorbic acid may aggravate stomach ulcers.
Long term use of ascorbic acid may deplete calcium, magnesium and potassium.
Vitamin C in the form of potassium ascorbate is contra-indicated in kidney disease.

Vitamin D / Calciferol

Please note that this information is indicative rather than comprehensive, serving as a reminder rather than a full explanation of the nature and role of this vitamin.

Fat-Soluble

Good Sources
Oily fish, oysters, egg yolks, offal, fortified margarine, blue cheese, cream.

Functions
Calcium and phosphorus metabolism (bone formation); heart action; nervous system maintenance.

Possible Deficiency Effects
Fatigue; spasms and twitching; hair loss; aching or weak bones; joint pains; muscle weakness; inadequate calcification of bones; skeletal deformity; delayed tooth eruption in babies; poor tooth enamel formation.

Possible Toxic Effects
Hypercalcaemia; renal stones; large deposits of calcium in body tissues; hypertension; excessive thirst; diarrhoea; poor appetite; nausea; weakness.

Intake
Upper safe limit for long-term use: 10 mcg per day.
UK RDA for pregnant and breastfeeding women and people confined indoors: 0.01 mg; no UK RDA for others.

Remarks
Lack of bile inhibits absorption from food and supplements.
Made in body when skin exposed to sunlight. The British Dietetic Association say: "It is estimated that in the UK ultraviolet light is only strong enough to make vitamin D on exposed skin in the middle of the day (probably about 10am - 3pm) during the summer months: April to September. Exposing skin for about 20 minutes (but longer for older people or those with darker skin) before applying sunscreen during these times, on most days, will probably ensure you make enough vitamin D to last you the whole year."

Low vitamin D levels have been linked to heart disease, diabetes and cancer, particularly in later life. An article in the Archives Of Internal Medicine (2007;167:1709-1710) reviewing studies involving more than 57,000 people shows that vitamin D supplements can reduce death rates by 7%.

The UK Foods Standard Agency recommends that older people, those who always cover their skin or rarely go outdoors, those who eat no meat or oily fish, and those of Asian origin should take 10 micrograms (0.01 mg, 400 i.u.) of vitamin D each day. The agency also recommends pregnant or breastfeeding women to take a vitamin D supplement.

The Canadian Cancer Society recommends that adults take a vitamin D supplement in fall and winter "due to our northern latitude and because the sun's rays are weak".

Supplements
Take with fatty food.
Absorption helped by calcium, phosphorus, vitamins E & C.
Avoid large intakes for any length of time; caution in individuals with kidney stones or a history of kidney stones.

Vitamin E / Tocopherols

Please note that this information is indicative rather than comprehensive, serving as a reminder rather than a full explanation of the nature and role of this vitamin.

Fat-Soluble

Good Sources
Vegetable oils, margarine, green vegetables, wheat germ, offal, eggs, corn, nuts, seeds, olives.

Functions
Protects membrane and red blood cells; inhibits coagulation of blood; protects fat-soluble vitamins; cellular respiration; works as an antioxidant (see page 99); helps the body use vitamin K (see page 158).

Possible Deficiency Effects
Increased risk of coronary heart disease and some cancers; acceleration of some degenerative diseases (e.g. cataracts, rheumatoid arthritis); acceleration of ageing; menopausal hot flushes; poor wound healing; haemolytic anaemia in babies.

Possible Toxic Effects
Raised blood pressure; minor gastrointestinal upsets.

Intake
Upper safe limit for long-term use: 800 mg per day.

Remarks
Antagonistic to vitamin K. Increases anti-coagulant effect of Warfarin, etc.
Iron reduces absorption of vitamin E.
Selenium may increase potency of E.
dl-alpha tocopherol, a synthetic form of vitamin E, is 50% less effective than natural d-alpha tocopherol.

Supplements
Take with fatty food. Absorption helped by selenium and vitamin C.
Absorption hindered by ferric iron and fried food.
Intake above 100 i.u. in individuals with high blood pressure should be used with caution.
Should not be taken with anticoagulant drugs or those with a recent history of heart disease unless supervised by a medical practitioner.
Women with hormonally dependent tumours should avoid high intakes in a base of wheat germ oil or other polyunsaturated oils.

Vitamin K

Please note that this information is indicative rather than comprehensive, serving as a reminder rather than a full explanation of the nature and role of this vitamin.

Fat-Soluble

Good Sources
Green leafy vegetables, fruits, cereals, dairy products, meat, soybeans.

Functions
Important in formation of blood clotting agents, involved in energy metabolism, protein formation in bone tissue.

Possible Deficiency Effects
Increased blood clotting time, osteoporosis; easily bruised skin; sore and bleeding gums; sluggish intestine; electrocardiogram abnormalities; haemorrhagic disease in newborn that can be fatal; some studies suggest that it helps promote strong bones in the elderly.

Possible Toxic Effects
Prolonged clotting time.

Intake
Upper safe limit for long-term use: not established.

Remarks
Vitamin K can be manufactured in the large intestine (see page 185). Broad-spectrum antibiotics destroy the gut flora that make vitamin K.

Appendix A2: Minerals

Boron

Please note that this information is indicative rather than comprehensive, serving as a reminder rather than a full explanation of the nature and role of this mineral.

Trace Mineral

Good Sources
Apples, pears, prunes, pulses, raisins, tomatoes

Functions
Thought to help the body make use of the glucose, fats, oestrogen and other minerals, such as calcium, copper and magnesium, in the food we eat.

Possible Deficiency Effects
Arthritis

Calcium

Please note that this information is indicative rather than comprehensive, serving as a reminder rather than a full explanation of the nature and role of this mineral.

Macromineral

Good Sources
Milk & milk products, fish, tofu, green vegetables, almonds, dried figs and dates.

Functions
Strong bones, teeth, muscle tissue; regulates heart beat, muscle action and nerve conduction; blood clotting.

Possible Deficiency Effects
Irregular heart beat; reduction in bone mass; increased risk of osteoporosis in later life; aching and weak bones; muscle cramps; twitching; joint pains; tingling hands and feet; nerve sensitivity; insomnia; chronic depression.

Possible Toxic Effects
Damage to the heart, liver and kidneys; constipation.

Intake
Upper safe limit for long-term use: 1500 mg per day.
UK RDA: 700 mg.

Remarks
Only about 30% consumed is absorbed; absorption reduced if shortage of vitamin D or low stomach acid.
A diet high in protein, sodium, sugar or caffeine can result in loss of calcium in the urine.

Supplements
Take with protein food or at bedtime.
Absorption helped by magnesium and vitamin D.
Absorption hindered by tea, coffee, smoking, phytic acid (page 70) in cereal grains particularly the bran, and excess iron.
Absorption hindered by inadequate hydrochloric acid in the stomach.

Chromium

Please note that this information is indicative rather than comprehensive, serving as a reminder rather than a full explanation of the nature and role of this mineral.

Trace Mineral

Good Sources
Brewers yeast, meat, whole grains, legumes, nuts, molasses.

Functions
Glucose metabolism; increases effectiveness of insulin. May be important for bone health, although research results not clear at the moment.

Possible Deficiency Effects
Diabetes; hypoglycaemia; alcohol intolerance; irritability; weakness.

Possible Toxic Effects
Lung disease.

Intake
No recommended intake, but levels of 50 to 200 mcg are generally regarded as safe. According to the US National Institutes of Health adult women in the United States consume about 23 to 29 mcg of chromium per day from food, and adult men average 39 to 54 mcg per day.

Remarks
Absorption rates from chromium in food very low – usually less than 2%.

Cobalt

Please note that this information is indicative rather than comprehensive, serving as a reminder rather than a full explanation of the nature and role of this mineral.

Trace Mineral

Good Sources
Fish, nuts, green leafy vegetables (such as broccoli and spinach), and cereals (such as oats).

Function
Major constituent of vitamin B12 (see page 149).

Possible Toxic Effects
May affect heart. May reduce fertility in men.

Copper

Please note that this information is indicative rather than comprehensive, serving as a reminder rather than a full explanation of the nature and role of this mineral.

Trace Mineral

Good Sources
Oysters, nuts, offal, legumes, parsley, molasses.

Functions
Formation of red blood cells; bone growth; works with vitamin C to form elastin.

Possible Deficiency Effects
Affects bone & blood formation & impair immune system in infants; depigmentation of the skin; possible role in cardiovascular disease; rheumatoid arthritis.

Possible Toxic Effects
Cardiovascular disease; possibly rheumatoid arthritis; (deficiency signs similar).

Intake
No RDA established, but adults are thought to need 1.5 to 3 mg of copper from food or supplementation per day. Copper excess is more common than copper deficiency.

Remarks
High intake of zinc or vitamin C over a long period may result in depletion of copper levels in the body.

Non-dietary sources include pesticides, fungicides, copper cooking utensils and some household water supplies. Use of the contraceptive pill can increase body copper levels.

Fluorine

Please note that this information is indicative rather than comprehensive, serving as a reminder rather than a full explanation of the nature and role of this mineral.

Trace Mineral

Good Sources
Some drinking water; fish; fluoride toothpaste.

Functions
Bone & tooth mineralisation.

Possible Deficiency Effects
Teeth that are susceptible to decay; lack of bone strength; possible increased risk of osteoporosis in later life.

Possible Toxic Effects
Mottling & crumbling of teeth; bone changes (fluorosis).

Intake
Upper safe limit for long-term use: not established.

Iodine

Please note that this information is indicative rather than comprehensive, serving as a reminder rather than a full explanation of the nature and role of this mineral.

Trace Mineral

Good Sources
Seafoods, sea salt, kelp. Amount in milk products and depends on the amount in the food supply of the cattle. Can be found in vegetables and fruit depending on the amount in the soil in which grown.

Function
Component of hormone thyroxine.

Possible Deficiency Effects
Goitre; lethargy; low metabolic rate; sensitivity to cold.

Possible Toxic Effects
Hyperthyroidism.

Intake
Adults need 0.14 mg a day; up to 0.5 mg a day unlikely to cause harm (UK Food Standards Agency).

Iron

Please note that this information is indicative rather than comprehensive, serving as a reminder rather than a full explanation of the nature and role of this mineral.

Trace Mineral

Good Sources
Lean meat & offal, fish, peas, leafy green vegetables, beans, treacle, lentils and haricot beans, almonds, dried apricots.

Functions
Haemoglobin formation; increases resistance to stress and disease; enzyme activity; formation of myoglobin (which carries oxygen) in muscles.

Possible Deficiency Effects
Anaemia; cracking at corner of mouth, recurrent mouth ulcers; sore tongue; poor hair growth; brittle nails; spoon-shaped (concave) nails; persistent tiredness; poor appetite; generalised itching; concentration problems; pale skin.

Possible Toxic Effects
Abdominal pain; arthritis; loss of libido; liver cancer.

Intake
Upper safe limit for long-term use: 15 mg per day.
UK RDA: 8.7 mg for men, and 14.8 mg for women.

Remarks
Haem iron derived from animal muscle or blood; non-haem iron is inorganic and more difficult to absorb; high intake of vitamin E, zinc, antacids, fibre and tea can interfere with absorption of non-haem iron; absorption enhanced by vitamin C and amino acids; 15% of intake is absorbed.

Supplements
Take with food.
Absorption helped by vitamin C.
Absorption hindered by tea, coffee, smoking, oxalic acid (in rhubarb etc.) phytic acid (see page 70) in cereal grains particularly the bran.
Absorption hindered by inadequate hydrochloric acid in the stomach.

Magnesium

Please note that this information is indicative rather than comprehensive, serving as a reminder rather than a full explanation of the nature and role of this mineral.

Macromineral

Good Sources
Nuts (particularly brazil nuts and almonds), green vegetables, whole grains, soya flour, peanuts, butter beans, treacle.

Functions
Acid/alkaline balance; important in metabolism of carbohydrates, minerals and sugar; bone structure; neuromuscular transmission.

Possible Deficiency Effects
Muscle weakness and cramps; twitching; irritability & tension; fatigue; headaches; concentration problems; premenstrual syndrome; apathy; poor appetite; diarrhoea; constipation; nausea and vomiting; irregular heart beats (arrhythmia).

Possible Toxic Effects
Muscle weakness; fatigue; sleepiness; hyper-excitability; diarrhoea.

Intake
Upper safe limit for long-term use: 300 mg per day.
UK RDA: 300 mg for men; 270 mg for women.

Remarks
Most common trace mineral deficiency in the developed world. 7 out of 10 women in the UK are reported as having inadequate intakes of this important mineral.

Supplements
Take with protein food or at bed time.
Absorption helped by calcium, vitamin D and vitamin B_6.
Absorption hindered by tea, coffee, smoking, and excess iron, and by inadequate hydrochloric acid in the stomach.

Manganese

Please note that this information is indicative rather than comprehensive, serving as a reminder rather than a full explanation of the nature and role of this mineral.

Trace Mineral

Good Sources
Tea (biggest source for many people), nuts, whole grains, fruits, vegetables.

Functions
Enzyme activation; carbohydrate & fat production; sex hormone production; skeletal development.

Possible Deficiency Effects
Joint pains; dizziness; schizophrenia.

Possible Toxic Effects
Lethargy; involuntary movements; impairment of voluntary movements; changes in muscle tone.

Intake
No RDAs set, but 1.8 mg per day for women and 2.3 mg per day for men is thought to be adequate.

Supplements
Take with protein food.
Absorption helped by vitamin C, and adequate hydrochloric acid in the stomach.
Absorption hindered by high doses of zinc, tea, coffee, smoking, and iron.
Older people tend to be more sensitive to the effect of manganese.

Molybdenum

Please note that this information is indicative rather than comprehensive, serving as a reminder rather than a full explanation of the nature and role of this mineral.

Trace Mineral

Good Sources
Beans, especially butter beans, buckwheat, lentils, liver and other organ meats, whole grains.

Function
Enzyme function particularly those involved in DNA metabolism.

Possible Deficiency Effects
Irritability; irregular heart beat; dental caries; male sexual impotence; cancer of the oesophagus; ankylosing spondilytis.

Possible Toxic Effects
Gout; increased urinary excretion of copper, joint pain.

Intake
US RDA is 45 mcg per day for adults.

Phosphorus

Please note that this information is indicative rather than comprehensive, serving as a reminder rather than a full explanation of the nature and role of this mineral.

Macromineral

Good Sources
Fish, meat, poultry, eggs, cereal, cereal products, brazil nuts, walnuts.

Functions
Bone development; important in protein, fat & carbohydrate utilisation.

Possible Deficiency Effects
Debility; loss of appetite; weakness; bone pain; tingling sensations; tremor; irritability; poor tooth enamel formation; sluggish intestine

Possible Toxic Effects
Prevents absorption of iron, calcium, magnesium & zinc; diarrhoea; calcification of soft tissues.

Intake
RDA is 550 mg per day. The average British diet includes between 1000 and 1500 mg of phosphorus on a daily basis.

Remarks
60% of intake absorbed; high phosphorus in unmodified cows milk a problem for babies.
High protein foods are high in phosphorus.
Colas and other soft drinks often contain high amounts of phosphorus.

Potassium

Please note that this information is indicative rather than comprehensive, serving as a reminder rather than a full explanation of the nature and role of this mineral.

Macromineral

Good Sources
Meat, vegetables, fruits, beans, dried peas, dried apricots and nuts

Functions
Fluid balance within cells; controls activity of heart muscle, nervous system & kidneys.

Possible Deficiency Effects
Muscle weakness; vomiting and diarrhoea; abdominal bloating; mental confusion; heart failure.

Possible Toxic Effects
Muscular weakness; mental apathy.

Intake
UK RDA: 3500 mg.

Selenium

Please note that this information is indicative rather than comprehensive, serving as a reminder rather than a full explanation of the nature and role of this mineral.

Trace Mineral

Good Sources
Seafood, offal, lean meat, eggs, whole grain.

Functions
Protects body tissues against oxidative radiation, pollution & normal metabolic by-products; works as an antioxidant (see page 99).

Possible Deficiency Effects
Muscle weakness; possible links with some forms of cancer & development of coronary heart disease; premature ageing.

Possible Toxic Effects
Dental caries; hair loss; skin depigmentation; abnormal nails; lassitude; gastrointestinal disturbances.

Intake
US RDA: 55 mcg per day for adults.

Sodium

Please note that this information is indicative rather than comprehensive, serving as a reminder rather than a full explanation of the nature and role of this mineral.

Macromineral

Good sources
Small amounts in many natural foods; high amounts in processed foods.

Function
Fluid balance of extra-cellular fluid; maintenance of acid-base balance; maintenance of blood pressure and blood volume; neuromuscular transmission.

Possible Deficiency Effects
Muscle cramps; fatigue; nausea.

Possible Toxic Effects
Hypertension; fluid retention.

Intake
Many people regularly exceed the recommended limit for dietary sodium, because of a high intake of salt (sodium chloride). The British Dietetic Association says: "The average salt intake is currently 9.5g a day (about 2 teaspoons), we should be having much less than this - the recommended intake is just 6g a day." These measurements take account of salt in processed food, etc., not just food you put on your meals.

Remarks
Sodium comprises 40% of common salt (sodium chloride); sea salt contains as much sodium as refined table salt.

Sulphur

Please note that this information is indicative rather than comprehensive, serving as a reminder rather than a full explanation of the nature and role of this mineral.

Macromineral

Good sources
Meat, fish, poultry, eggs, cheese, beans.

Function
Constituent of hormones, collagen, insulin, thiamine & biotin; regulates various body activities.

Possible Deficiency Effects
Skin & hair problems.

Vanadium

Please note that this information is indicative rather than comprehensive, serving as a reminder rather than a full explanation of the nature and role of this mineral.

Trace Mineral

Good sources
Parsley, lobster, radishes, dill.

Function
Fat metabolism.

Possible Deficiency Effects
Bipolar disorder, ankylosing spondilytis

Possible Toxic Effects
Stomach cramps and diarrhoea; greenish coloured tongue.

Remarks
Excess removed by vitamin C.

Zinc

Please note that this information is indicative rather than comprehensive, serving as a reminder rather than a full explanation of the nature and role of this mineral.

Trace Mineral

Good Sources
Lean meat, liver, eggs, cheese, seafood (particularly oysters), whole grains, sesame seeds, walnuts, brazil nuts, lentils.

Functions
Involved in digestion & metabolism; important in development of reproductive system; wound healing; insulin production; growth.

Possible Deficiency Effects
Persistent leg ulcers & pressure sores; poor wound healing; red, greasy skin on face; scaly dry flaky skin; eczema; dermatitis; poor hair growth and hair loss; dandruff; night blindness; brittle nails; white spots on nails; poor appetite; diarrhoea; irritability; depression; growth retardation.

Possible Toxic Effects
Impaired iron & copper absorption; suppressed immune system; gastrointestinal disturbances.

Intake
Upper safe limit for long-term use: 15 mg per day.
UK RDA: 5.5 mg to 9.5 mg for men and 4mg to 7 mg for women.

Remarks
Antagonistic to copper.
Increased requirement in women taking the contraceptive pill.

Supplements
Take with food or at bedtime.
Absorption helped by vitamin C and vitamin B_6
Absorption hindered by lead, copper, calcium, tea, coffee, alcohol, excess iron, phytic acid in cereal grains particularly the bran.
Absorption hindered by inadequate hydrochloric acid in the stomach.

Appendix B1: Food Classifications - Culinary

This can be done in various ways. Here is one possibility:

Meat

Fish

Dairy

Chicken and eggs
Vegetables

Herbs

Pulses
Pasta and rice

Fruit

Seeds and nuts

Oils and fats

Spices

Bread, cakes

Processed food

Other

Appendix B2: Food Classifications - Nutritional

Proteins/amino acids

Fats

Carbohydrate

Vitamins

Minerals

Fibre

Phytochemicals

Other

Appendix B3: Food Classifications - Botanical

Plants

Fungi or moulds
Baker's yeast (hence breads and doughs, etc.), Brewer's yeast (hence alcoholic beverages), mushroom, truffle, chanterelle, cheese, vinegar (hence pickles and sauces).

Grasses
Wheat, corn, barley, oats, millet, cane sugar, bamboo shoots, rice, rye. (Note that buckwheat is *not* a member of the grass family.)

Lily
Onion, asparagus, chives, leek, garlic, sarsaparilla, shallot.

Mustard
Broccoli, cabbage, cauliflower, Brussels sprouts, horse-radish, kohlrabi, radish, swede, turnip, watercress, mustard and cress.

Rose
Apple, pear, quince, almond, apricot, cherry, peach, plum, sloe, blackberry, loganberry, raspberry, strawberry.

Pulses or Legumes
Pea, chick pea, soy bean (hence TVP), lentils, liquorice, peanut, kidney bean, string bean, haricot bean, mung bean, alfalfa.

Citrus
Orange, lemon, grapefruit, tangerine, clementine, ugly, Satsuma, lime.

Cashew
Cashew nut, mango, pistachio (also poison ivy).

Grape
Wine, champagne, brandy, sherry, raisin, currant, sultana, cream of tartar.

Parsley
Carrot, parsley, dill, celery, fennel, parsnip, aniseed.

Nightshade
Potato, tomato, tobacco, aubergine, pepper (chilli, paprika).

Gourd
Honeydew melon, watermelon, cucumber, squashes, cantaloupe, gherkin, courgette, pumpkin.

Composite
Lettuce, chicory, sunflower, safflower, burdock, dandelion, camomile, artichoke, pyrethrum.

Mint
Mint, basil, marjoram, oregano, sage, rosemary, thyme.

Palm
Coconut, date, sago.

Walnut
Walnut, pecan.

Goosefoot
Spinach, chard, sugar beet.

Sterculia
Chocolate (cacao bean), cocoa, cola nut.

The following commonly eaten plants have no *commonly* eaten relatives: juniper, pineapple, yam, banana, vanilla (often a chemical imitation), black pepper, hazelnut, chestnut, fig, avocado, maple, lychee, kiwi fruit, tea, coffee, papaya, brazil nut, ginseng, olive, sweet potato, sesame (also as tahini).

Animals

Bovines
Cattle (beef), milk and dairy products, mutton, lamb, goat.

Poultry
Chicken, eggs, pheasant, quail, (not turkey).

Duck
Duck, goose.

Swine
Pork, bacon, lard (dripping), ham, sausage, pork scratchings.

Flatfish
Dab, flounder, halibut, turbot, sole, plaice.

Salmon
Salmon, trout.

Mackerel
Tuna, bonito, tuny, mackerel, skipjack

Codfish
Haddock, cod, ling (saith), coley, hake.

Herring
Pilchard, sardine, herring, rollmop.
Molluscs
Snail, abalone, squid, clam, mussel, oyster, scallop.

Crustaceans
Lobster, prawn, shrimp, crab, crayfish.

The following commonly eaten animals and fishes have no *commonly* eaten relatives: anchovy, sturgeon (caviar), whitefish, turkey, rabbit, deer (venison).

This information is taken from:

The Food Allergy Plan Dr Keith Mumby, Unwin Paperbacks, ISBN 0 04 641047 3

Appendix C: The Digestive System

The digestive system is concerned with the breakdown and absorption of food and the excretion of waste. Enzymes are responsible for speeding up or slowing down chemical reactions.

The Mouth, Salivary Glands And Teeth

Summary: This is where the food first enters the body. Food is broken down physically. Some carbohydrate digestion occurs in the mouth.

There are 3 pairs of salivary glands:

- Parotid
- Submandibular
- Sublingual

These glands secrete saliva, which contains the enzyme ptyalin (also called salivary amylase) that changes carbohydrates into maltose and dextrin. The water in the saliva starts the process of dissolving the food. The enzyme lysozyme destroys bacteria and so helps prevent tooth decay.

Proper chewing is important in order to prepare the food for digestion further down the alimentary canal. Chewing physically breaks down the food and also ensures that saliva is thoroughly mixed with it.

The Pharynx & Oesophagus

The food passes over the closed entrance to the larynx and through the pharynx into the oesophagus. The food moves down the oesophagus by peristaltic action (see under large intestine). The food takes approximately 9 seconds to be moved from the pharynx to the stomach.

The Stomach

Summary: In the stomach food is mixed with the gastric juices. Proteins are converted to peptones through the action of pepsin.

The cardiac sphincter prevents food going back into the oesophagus. In the stomach the food is churned up and mixed with gastric juices that are secreted by the gastric glands. This mixture is referred to as chyme. The stomach contains:

- Mucus cells that secrete a special mucus that protects the stomach lining from the effect of the gastric juices.

- Chief cells that secrete the enzyme pepsinogen. Pepsinogen is converted by hydrochloric acid into the enzyme pepsin. Pepsin turns proteins into peptones. In children rennin is also secreted here. Rennin turns milk protein into casein, which allows pepsin to act upon it.

- Oxyntic cells that secrete hydrochloric acid. Hydrochloric acid produces the acid environment required by the gastric enzymes, kills bacteria, stops the action of ptyalin, converts pepsinogen into pepsin and controls the pylorus. Intrinsic factor is also secreted which is involved in the absorption of Vitamin B12.

The gastric glands automatically secrete gastric juices when food is present, but the stomach also produces the hormone gastrin, which passes into the blood and stimulates the production of gastric juices when it reaches the gastric glands.

Food stays in the stomach for between 0.5 and 3 hours in general. If the meal is mainly carbohydrate with very little protein it will leave the stomach in about 0.5 hours. Fat rich food stays in the stomach for the longest time.

The Small Intestine
Summary: This is the main organ of digestion. Complex sugars are turned into simpler sugars. Fats are turned into fatty acids and glycerol. Peptones (from proteins) are turned into amino acids. The nutrients are then absorbed through the wall of the small intestine.

The opening to the small intestine is through the pylorus. When the food in the stomach reaches the correct degree of acidity in the area next to the pylorus, the pyloric sphincter opens to allow some of the food into the small intestine. Acid levels in the digestive tract are affected by stress, so stress can have a big affect on nutrient absorption and waste excretion.

Food is digested and absorbed through the wall of the small intestine. Villi increase the surface area of the small intestine.

At the end of the small intestine is the ileo-caecal valve, which controls the entry of the chyme into the large intestine.

The small intestine is divided into:

- The duodenum
- The jejunum
- The ileum

3 hormones are secreted in the duodenum to ensure proper sequence of digestion:

- Secretin
- Cholecystokinin (CCK)
- Gastric inhibitory peptide

The gall bladder and liver are connected to the duodenum by ducts. Lymphatic nodes deal with any bacteria absorbed with the food.

Digestion is carried out by:

- Pancreatic juices (containing trypsinogen, amylase, lipase and sodium bicarbonate)
- Bile from the liver and gall bladder
- Intestinal juices

The intestinal juices are secreted in response to the food and also to the hormone secretin (produced in intestine). The intestinal juices contain enzymes: enterokinase, peptidase, maltase, sucrase, lactase and lipase. These are mixed with the food by peristalsis.

The enzymes change peptones (from proteins) into amino acids and convert complex sugars into simple sugars (e.g. glucose). These are then absorbed through the intestinal wall into the blood stream.

The bile and the juices emulsify fats. Lipase converts fats into fatty acids and glycerol, which are water-soluble. These are absorbed through the intestinal wall and transported via the lymph system into the blood stream.

Water is absorbed passively as a result of sodium being actively absorbed.

Most vitamins and minerals diffuse through the small intestine walls, but some have an active carrier mechanism (e.g. iron is taken into the cells by carrier proteins).

The Large Intestine

Summary: Absorption of water and salts takes place here. Fermentation of carbohydrate and production of some vitamins.

The food remains in the large intestine for 3-10 hours usually. Water and salts are absorbed and faeces are excreted via the anus. Some B vitamins and Vitamin K are also produced as a by-product of normal bacterial activity and are absorbed through the colon wall. Any remaining carbohydrates are fermented here through the action of the gut bacteria.

The movement of the solids through the bowel is controlled by peristaltic action. In peristalsis muscles contract and dilate rhythmically allowing food to pass through them. The parasympathetic nervous system increases the rate and the sympathetic nervous system reduces it. Peristalsis occurs less frequently here than in the small intestine and oesophagus.

The Liver
The liver has many functions. These include:

- Breaking down stored fat to produce energy.
- Converting excess amino acids into urea.
- Destroying worn-out bloods cells.
- Detoxifying drugs and poisons.
- Chemically altering hormones such as thyroxine.
- Synthesising vitamin A from carotene.
- Converting excess carbohydrate into fat for storage and producing bile: bile aids in the digestion of fats.

The Gall Bladder
The gall bladder acts as a storage place for the bile produced by the liver. When necessary it concentrates and stores the bile. Cholecystokinin, a hormone produced in the mucosa of the small intestine, stimulates the release of the bile when fats enter the small intestine.

The Pancreas
The pancreas is part of the endocrine and the digestive system as it produces both hormones (e.g. glucagon and insulin) and digestive enzymes (e.g. amylase).

Glucagon and insulin help to control blood sugar levels. Glucagon stimulates the conversion of glycogen into glucose and so raises blood sugar levels.

Insulin lowers blood sugar levels by stimulating the conversion of glucose into glycogen, which can then be stored until needed, and also by allowing glucose to enter cells through special glucose channels. This table summarises this:

Hormone	Affects	Blood Sugar
Glucagon	Turns glycogen into glucose for use	Raises blood sugar
Insulin	Turns glucose into glycogen for storage Allows glucose to enter cells	Decreases blood sugar

The pancreas produces pancreatic juices (see under small intestine). These juices are slightly alkaline and so stop the action of pepsin. They create the proper medium for the enzymes in the small intestine.

Appendix D1: Life Stage Considerations

Pregnancy

Dietary advice needs to consider both the needs of the mother and the foetus.

Early on in the pregnancy it is the baby that will suffer most from any nutritional inadequacies in the mother's diet.

As pregnancy progresses the nutritional demands of the foetus take precedence over those of the mother, so it is the mother rather than the baby who will suffer if the mother's diet is inadequate.

During pregnancy adaptive mechanisms occur in the mother to increase maternal absorption of vitamins and minerals and decrease their excretion. Protein and energy metabolism becomes more efficient also and nutrient stores are mobilised. Good pre-conceptual nutrition for both the prospective parents is now being seen as also important to the future health of the baby.

- Calories: on average an extra 200 kcal/day are needed in the final third of pregnancy
- Protein: usually existing protein intake is enough to meet the extra requirements of pregnancy.
- Folic acid: chronic folate deficiency can result in spina bifida and related problems. The need for folate is from very early on in the pregnancy, so women are now advised to eat folate rich foods or take a folate supplement (0.4 mg/day) for the first 12 weeks of pregnancy and ideally before conception. Women who have already had a foetus with spina bifida etc. are advised to take 5.0 mg of folate per day. Folate containing foods include dark green leafy vegetables, pulses and fortified breakfast cereals.
- Iron: no dietary increase is necessary; the extra required is met from cessation of periods, increased absorption and mobilisation of reserves.
- Vitamin D: increased needs mean that a supplement of 10 mcg per day are recommended where exposure to sunlight is not sufficient.
- Vitamin C: intake should be increased.
- Alcohol: alcohol should probably be avoided completely during the first three months and only in moderation after that.
- Vitamin A: animal experiments have shown that excessive intake (more than 6000 mcg/day) can cause foetal abnormalities, so caution in supplementation is advised. It is advised that liver (a rich source of vitamin A) should be avoided for this reason.

Lactation

During breastfeeding women have increased nutrient needs.

- Calories: on average an additional 500 kcal/day which may be derived from adipose tissue (fat) laid down during pregnancy.

- Fluid: fluid intake increased to compensate for the amount in breast milk.

- Protein, calcium, folate, vitamin C, vitamin A: requirements increase.

- Caffeine and alcohol: excreted in the breast milk so should be avoided.

- Allergens: where the baby has an allergic reaction to a food this will often occur also if the mother eats the food. Food proteins (the most likely source of an allergen in a food) are known to pass into breast milk.

Infants

The quality of nutrition in infancy has long-term consequences and may affect susceptibility to diseases such as coronary heart disease in later life.

There are two main considerations:

- Energy and nutrient needs are high.

- Many of the baby's body systems are relatively immature, so inappropriate feeding can cause problems.

Breast milk is the best start for the baby. Advantages include:

- Ideal nutritional composition.

- Nutrient composition changes along with development of the baby.

- Protects against infection by providing antibodies.

- Bacteriologically safe, so no issues of sterilisation and bacterial contamination.

- May help mother lose excess adipose tissue associated with pregnancy.

If the mother is HIV positive or taking certain drugs, breast-feeding may not be appropriate.

Lactose intolerance occurs when a baby is deficient in the enzyme lactase. Symptoms include explosive, frothy diarrhoea, abdominal cramps and vomiting. Babies can have problems with cow's milk for reasons other than lactose intolerance.

Weaning

Weaning should be a gradual process starting not earlier than 6 months of age. Earlier weaning is inappropriate because of the immaturity of many organs.

Foods that are high in salt, sugar, fibre or have had their fat content reduced (e.g. skimmed milk) are not suitable weaning foods.

Eggs, cows milk, wheat, peanuts and citrus fruit should be introduced with caution as they are common allergens Small babies should not be given whole nuts or other foods where there is a possibility of choking.

Elderly People

The requirements for energy (calories) usually decline with age as people become less active, but the requirements for protein, vitamins and minerals remain the same. This means that the diet needs to be nutrient dense. Absorption is often poorer than in younger people too. Problems with chewing can limit absorption further.

Medication can interfere directly with absorption of nutrients. In addition side effects (e.g. loss of appetite and nausea) can lead to reluctance to eat. Lack of money, reduced mobility leading to shopping difficulties and problems with manual dexterity can also lead to an impoverished diet.

- Fats: lower (or maintain low levels) total consumption of all fats in general and saturated fats in particular.

- Salt: high salt intake increases the risk of hypertension.

- Iron: absorption tends to be poor and many drugs interfere with its absorption.

- Zinc: important in wound healing. (Leg ulcers and pressure sores may respond to increasing zinc levels.)

- Calcium: low calcium levels will exacerbate problems of loss of bone density (osteoporosis).

- Vitamin D: main source is sunlight, but this may be limited for elderly people. Vitamin D supplementation is likely to be necessary for those who are housebound.

- Folate and vitamin B12: absorption often low so megaloblastic anaemia can result.

Appendix D2: Interactions Between Medication, Food And Supplements

The information in this section needs to be dealt with appropriately. In many countries it is illegal to suggest that someone deviates from their doctor's instructions.

- Cause gastric irritation, e.g. aspirin and non-steroidal anti-inflammatory drugs should be taken with food to minimise this problem.

- Change gastrointestinal pH, e.g. antacids neutralise stomach acids and so reduce vitamin B12 absorption.

- Change gastrointestinal motility, so that food moves faster or more slowly through the intestines, e.g. laxatives speed the transition time; aluminium, which is in many antacids, has a relaxing effect on some muscles and so delays gastric emptying time.

- Form insoluble complexes with components of food; this means that neither the drug nor the nutrient (usually a mineral) will be absorbed, e.g. tetracyclines bind to calcium in dairy products.

- Affect nutrient metabolism and distribution, e.g. anticonvulsive drugs affect folic acid metabolism; aspirin competes with folate for binding-sites on serum proteins.

- Affect nutrient excretion, e.g. corticosteroids increase excretion of potassium and increase retention of sodium; diuretics may increase the excretion of potassium, magnesium, calcium and the water-soluble vitamins.

- Affect bowel flora, e.g. antibiotics can lead to a reduction of the beneficial bacteria in the gut that produce vitamin K.

- Side effects that either increase or decrease appetite, e.g. anticonvulsant drugs can cause diarrhoea and reduce appetite.

- Not understood effects, e.g. aspirin has been reported to lower plasma vitamin C concentrations, but how it does this is not known.

- Steroid drugs have the potential to interfere with the absorption and utilisation of calcium, potassium, sodium, protein, and vitamins C and D.

Effect Of Food On Drugs

Some foods affect drug absorption and use. This is usually set out in the leaflet that comes with the drug. Examples include:

- Garlic can affect anticoagulants and diabetes medication.
- Ginkgo biloba can affect anticoagulant medication.
- Grapefruit can cause the body to absorb more of some drugs such as antihistamines, statins, benzodiazepines.
- St John's Wort (a herbal supplement) may affect the contraceptive pill and the antidepressant Prozac.
- Alcohol interacts with some drugs particularly those that have an effect on the brain, e.g. sleeping pills, antidepressants.
- Over-ripe cheese, pickles, some beers and red wine can affect MAO antidepressants, leading to a dangerous rise in blood pressure.
- Cranberry juice can affect Warfarin.

Diabetus Mellitus

High doses of Vitamin C can cause problems with glucose monitoring tests.

Renal Failure

Patients with renal failure should not take doses of calcium exceeding 1 gm per day because of the risk of hypercalcaemia or potassium doses exceeding 500 mg per dose because of the risk of hyperkalaemia.

Thyroid Disorders

Iodine can affect the functioning of the thyroid, and should only be taken under medical supervision.

Appendix D3: Reactive Hypoglycaemia

The islets of Langerhans in the pancreas produce insulin. As blood-sugar levels rise, the insulin travels to the liver and the muscles instructing them to take glucose from the blood stream and to store it as glycogen. When blood-sugar levels start to drop, the pancreas releases glucagon. This stimulates the breakdown of the stores of glycogen and their release back into the bloodstream as glucose. The effects of glucagon and insulin are opposing: between them they are usually able to keep blood-sugar levels stable.

Hormone	Affects	Blood Sugar
Glucagon	Turns glycogen into glucose for use	Raises blood sugar
Insulin	Turns glucose into glycogen for storage Allows glucose to enter cells	Decreases blood sugar

The liver releases a substance called glucose tolerance factor. This is thought to be composed of three amino acids (glycine, glutamic acid and cysteine), plus chromium and vitamin B_3. This aids glucose uptake by the target cells. The hormones adrenaline and the gluco-corticoids are released by the adrenal glands in response to stress. These also raise the blood-sugar levels by stimulating the pancreas and the liver. If blood-sugar levels are low, the hypothalamus is stimulated and hunger is experienced.

The ideal is for blood sugar levels to remain more or less constant with a slight peak after eating and dropping slightly as the person experiences hunger. When people are suffering from reactive hypoglycaemia, they experience rapid rises in blood sugar following eating and then the blood sugar level drops rapidly. This usually results in symptoms such as mood swings, headaches, trembling, palpitations, sweating, excessive hunger, and craving for sweet foods. While eating foods high in sugar will often temporarily alleviate symptoms, in the long run this further exacerbates the problem. Reactive hypoglycaemia will often develop as a result of a diet high in foods with a high glycaemic index (see page 63). These enter the blood stream rapidly and can, over time, upset the insulin-glucagon balance.

There are various strategies that can help people who suffer from hypoglycaemia. The correct one or combination can be established through testing:

- Eating food with a low glycaemic index (see page 63).
- Reducing/ eliminating alcohol.
- Supplementing with amino acids, vitamin B_3 and chromium.
- Eating little and often – but not increasing the amount eaten overall (see page 50).
- Checking for food allergies - allergy reactions can lead to swings in blood sugar levels.
- Reducing stress levels.
- Using energy work to correct any hormonal imbalances etc.

Appendix D4: Obesity & Weight Problems

The number of adipose cells increases between birth and two years of age. It is then relatively stable until puberty when the number increases further as a result of hormonal activity. After this the number of fat cells does not increase. The size of the cells will increase if the individual becomes obese.

There appears to be two sorts of body fat:

- Ordinary subcutaneous fat that is mainly to store energy.

- Brown fat that burns up excess energy and provides heat.

There are suggestions that some obese individuals have relatively inactive brown fat. It has also been suggested that this inactivity of brown fat may be due to nutritional deficiencies.

Functions Of Adipose Tissue
Adipose tissue (body fat):

- Insulates against heat loss.

- Provides protective cushioning around organs.

- Produces hormones such as leptin (see page 197), resistin, adiponectin, interleukin-6 and tumour necrosis factor alpha, which have important roles in the body.

- Provides an emergency reserve of energy.

Body Mass Index
This is a method of assessing how over weight someone is:

BMI = Weight (measured in kilograms) divided by height squared (measured in metres)

e.g. BMI = 78kg ÷ [1.79m x 1.79m] =24.3

Canadian and US equivalent:

$$BMI = Weight \text{ (measured in pounds)} \times 703 \text{ divided by height squared}$$
(measured in inches)

Height is measured without shoes. Weight is measured without shoes and in indoor clothing.

Body Mass Index	Classification
< 20	underweight
20 - 24.9	grade 0 - normal
25 - 29.9	grade 1 - overweight
30-40	grade 2 - obesity
> 40	grade 3 - severe obesity

In the U.K. approximately a quarter of the adult population is classed as obese, and in the USA a third of adults are.

Waist-Hip Ratio (WHR)
The area where the fat is deposited is significant in terms of risk of certain diseases. Central obesity where the fat occurs in and around the abdomen increases the risk of the person developing diabetes and coronary heart disease.

WHR= waist circumference (cms) ÷ hip circumference (cms)

Obesity accompanied by a high WHR (greater than 0.9 in men and 0.8 in women) is associated with an increased risk of cardiovascular disease.

Putting it another way: a quick rule of thumb is that men with a waist measurement of more than 100 cms (40 inches) and women with a waist measurement of more than 87.5 cms (35 inches) are at a much greater risk of these illnesses than other people.

The reason for this is that fat cells around the stomach pump out proteins and hormones that can trigger insulin resistance, with the resulting adverse effect on your health.

Health Problems Of Obesity
There are many health problems associated with obesity. Obese people have:

- An increased risk of cardiovascular disease.

- Reduced life expectancy.

- Increased blood pressure.

- Elevated cholesterol.

- A reduced ability to take exercise and manage every day tasks.

- Increased risk of gallstones.

- Increased risk of diabetes and diabetic retinopathy. Obese women are almost 13 times more likely to develop Type 2 Diabetes than non-obese women. The figure for men is times as likely.

- Age-related macular degeneration (AMD) of the eyes.

- Cataracts (the risk of developing cataracts for obese people can be as high as double that of people who are not overweight).

- Increased risk of varicose veins.

- Increased risk of hiatus hernia.

- Increased risk of constipation.

- Increased risk of post-operative infections.

- Poor wound healing.

- Increased risk of osteoarthritis.

- Back problems.

And for women additionally:

- An increased risk of irregular periods and period pains.

- An increased risk of hairiness and cancers of the breast and womb.

The health risks increase if one or both parents are over-weight.

Positive benefits of obesity include a reduced risk of osteoporosis and an increased tolerance of cold weather.

Possible Reasons For Being Overweight
This is often a complex issue and not all interventions are within the remit of nutritional work.

- Heavy reliance on high calorie convenience foods. (See page 112.)

- Inappropriate food choices.

- Inappropriate eating habits triggered by stress, anxiety, boredom, etc.

- Eating too much overall. (See page 59.)

- Too little exercise: a good exercise programme has been shown repeatedly to be one of the best ways of losing weight.

- Low metabolic rate.

- Constant dieting affecting metabolic rates (a diet of less than 1000 calories a day can lead the body to adapt to a famine situation and slow down the metabolic rate by as much as 40%).

- Clinical disease, e.g. under-active thyroid.

- Cravings – see page 199.

- Lack of protein – protein (page 71) gives a sense of fullness and also helps to keep up the metabolic rate.

- Allergies can directly affect the thyroid.

- Constant hunger caused by the body "searching" for nutrients it is deficient in.

- There is a theory, substantially unproved, that fat deposits are a relatively harmless place to store toxins, so that the body will not release the fat because it also means releasing the toxins, which could damage vital organs when they enter the blood stream.

- The person misreads body signs of thirst for hunger, and so eats when should be drinking water. (See page 65.)

- Eating too quickly so that mind does not register the replete sensation till it is too late (see page 43)

- Hormone problems: Recent research has identified the hormone leptin as a central player in the control of appetite (possibly via its effect on neuropeptide Y). Leptin is produced by the fat cells when there is fat in them. The leptin travels via the blood stream to the hypothalamus where it moderates appetite. The fatter the person is the higher the levels of leptin there are circulating in the blood. It appears that in overweight people the brain is in some way insensitive to the message of the leptin. Over weight people may also have problems with other hormones, e.g. GLP1, orexins, somatastatin, CART, etc. Energy procedures can often be used to correct these problems.

Atkins Diet

Popular as a weight loss diet, relying on protein, fat and a limited amount of salad and vegetables and 8 glasses of water a day.
Severely restricts carbohydrate, caffeine and alcohol.
Nuts, seeds and berries are usually added after the induction phase.

The diet works by inducing a state of ketosis in the body. In ketosis the body produces ketones (similar to acetone, which is a solvent found in nail varnish). In ketosis the body is unable to use glucose as its energy source, and is forced to use fat instead. Fatty acids are released into the blood, and these are turned into ketones.

There is a lot of evidence that the Atkins diet works in the early stages, but some of the initial weight loss is due to loss of water rather than fat. Like other diets it has a high drop out rate, because of how restrictive it is. There are concerns about the long-term effect of this diet, as it is low in minerals and vitamins and high in saturated fat.

There is good information on this and other diets at www.dieting-review.com.

Underweight Problems

In the extreme form this can result in anorexia and bulimia. One of the best ways to put on weight may be by alternately dieting and eating a lot. When a person goes on a diet, the body senses that a famine may ensue and so takes measures to conserve fat by, for example, reducing the metabolic rate. When the person starts eating more, the metabolic rate does not immediately increase. Underweight people can sometimes use this effectively to reduce their metabolic rate.

Possible Reasons For Being Underweight

- Zinc deficiency: zinc is important for sense of smell and taste, and so may affect appetite.
- Psychological problems such as an unwillingness to be in the world, or conflict over attaining adulthood.
- Problems with nutrient absorption.
- Clinical disease, e.g. coeliac disease, over-active thyroid, Crohn's disease, etc.

Appendix D5: Cravings

There are four main reasons for food cravings:

- Nutrient deficiencies
- Allergies
- Blood sugar problems
- Emotional associations

Nutrient Deficiencies

Craving particular foods can be a sign of a need for a nutrient that is in the food that is craved, e.g. a deficiency of potassium may result in a craving for avocados and bananas, and a shortage of zinc may stimulate a desire for sunflower seeds and oysters.

When there was lead in petrol, I found that a lot of clients who had a problem with lead loved apples. These are an excellent source of pectin, which helps to remove lead from the body. You may know little about nutrition, but instinctively your body is trying to do the right thing.

Allergy Induced Cravings

Allergy induced cravings leading to bingeing and inappropriate eating patterns. The key to understanding this may be down to endorphins, chemicals produced by the body that inhibit pain, and which are at least partially responsible for the "runner's high" and the phenomenon of soldiers continuing to fight even when severely injured. Endorphins are the body's own morphine. (In fact the term "endorphin" is derived from "endogenous morphine", i.e. morphine produced within the body.)

Although it is not totally clear why you may become addicted to your allergen, endorphins and food particles that mimic endorphins are likely to be involved. Several studies have shown that endorphin production increases during allergic reactions. In addition, protein fragments called exorphins may be formed when food is broken down. These were first named and described in 1979 by Zioudro, Streaty and Klee. These can act like endorphins in the body. It is believed that if you are an allergy sufferer your body becomes adapted to that higher level of endorphin activity and so craves the allergen in order to maintain the endorphin levels.

The allergy-addiction link may also throw light on why you find it impossible to stick to a diet, developing seemingly irresistible cravings that you feel unable to control. There are two possible scenarios. You could be allergic to some high calorie food such as chocolate or crisps and find it extremely difficult to moderate your consumption because you are addicted to it. You follow your diet but the urge to eat the allergen becomes greater and greater until you can resist it no longer - like a drug addict you are reaching for your fix. You stuff the food down, almost without tasting it, desperately trying to turn off the craving as quickly as possible. As calm returns you realise just how much you have eaten and feel depressed and guilty. This can then lead to another round of eating as you feel that having broken the diet you may as well continue eating.

The other possibility is that you experience cravings, but for some reason do not connect the withdrawal symptoms with a particular food. In this case, as you start to feel "hungry" you keep on eating different foods without feeling satisfied. You only stop when you consume the addictive allergen. Overall calorie consumption can be very high even if the allergen is to a low calorie food such as lettuce, because of all the other food that is eaten without satisfying the "hungry" feeling before you get to the lettuce.

Blood Sugar Swings

It is important for health that blood sugar levels stay within reasonable limits. This is taken care of by two hormones – glucagon and insulin. (See page 192 for more information on this.) Most of the time this works fine, but sometimes blood sugar levels can drop. Low blood sugar has a very detrimental effect on the functioning of the brain. As this can threaten your survival, low blood sugar is treated by the body as an emergency situation. When blood sugar drops suddenly, a primitive reflex tells you to eat immediately. It is difficult to ignore this command, and in general you eat whatever happens to be handy and is sufficiently rich in carbohydrate. This is not necessarily nutritious food. Other signs of badly fluctuating blood sugar levels include headaches, trembling, panic attacks, sudden sweating and anxiety.

The main strategies for dealing with this are:

- Avoiding high glycaemic index food. High glycaemic foods cause the blood sugar level to increase suddenly and then drop steeply. Avoiding high glycaemic index food can help to stabilise blood sugar. Adding just one low GI food item to each meal has been shown to have a positive effect on blood sugar levels, according to a study published in the February 2005 edition of the *British Journal of Nutrition*.

- Ensuring an adequate supply of nutrients that affect blood sugar levels. Chromium (see page 161), a trace mineral, can help the body use insulin more effectively, and can help stabilise blood sugar. Good food sources of chromium include brewers yeast, whole grains, legumes, nuts and molasses., but if your blood sugar is very erratic you would probably do better to take a chromium supplement.

Emotional Associations

Many people find that when they are ill they crave a particular food or meal, because that is what their mother gave to them when they were ill as a child. If your client was given a bar of chocolate every time something very stressful happened as a child, or as a reward for good behaviour, it is likely to be a powerful pull.

These are not mutually exclusive. Your client could crave walnuts for their balance of essential fatty acids, and cakes to counteract a blood sugar swing.

Appendix D6: Candidiasis

Common symptoms are:

- Rectal and vaginal itching
- Nausea
- Abdominal bloating
- Irritable bowel and intestinal gas
- Many other symptoms (including fatigue, eczema, post-viral syndrome, joint swelling, asthma and allergies) have been associated with the problem.

The symptoms are the result of an overgrowth of the common yeast Candida albicans. The candida organism is normally present in the bowel of most people, and is held in check by the ecological balance between the various gut flora. The natural antagonist of candida is lactobacillus acidophilus.

Factors that allow the overgrowth to occur include:

- A diet high in refined carbohydrate (particularly white sugar)
- Frequent use of certain drugs (e.g. antibiotics, steroids and oral contraceptives)

It is believed that the candida can change from a yeast to a fungal form when conditions are favourable. This can lead to a breakdown in the integrity of the intestinal tract, which then allows incompletely digested proteins and candida organisms into the bloodstream. Candida albicans also releases toxins that affect the immune system. A self-diagnosis of candida problems is very popular at the moment. Treatment often involves extreme diets. Even where this works this does *not necessarily* prove that candida is a problem, as the diet excludes so much it could be the removal of an allergen which leads to the improvement.

Nutritional treatment of candida:

- Following a low sugar, highly nutritious diet
- Garlic, caprylic acid, pau d'arco tea and probiotics (in yoghurt and supplements) have been found helpful against candida.
- Colon cleansing: using herbs (e.g. psyllium husks), colonics etc.

Appendix E: Food Safety Guidelines

Food Safety

Many problems of food safety arise either from faulty storage of food (usually in the home) or incorrect preparation of food.

Food poisoning can be caused by bacteria, bacterial toxins, viruses, mycotoxins from moulds and fungi, chemical toxins (e.g. undercooked kidney beans) or protozoa.

- **Gastro-intestinal symptoms** can be caused by salmonella, campylobacter, staphylococci, escherichia coli (E. coli), shigella, enteroviruses, rotaviruses and parvoviruses.
- **Flu-like symptoms** can be caused by listeria (particularly a problem for pregnant women) and toxoplasmosis.
- **Neurological symptoms** can be caused by clostridium botulinum (extremely rare) and neurotoxins present in some undercooked beans.

General Food Safety Guidelines

It is important to protect food from contamination, cook properly and store appropriately.

Appropriate measures include:

- Covering food to avoid flies etc.
- Washing hands before handling food.
- Keeping pets' food and drink bowls separate from those for humans.
- Keeping pets away from food and kitchen surfaces.
- Keeping kitchen surfaces, etc. clean.
- Keeping different types of food separate from each other, particularly raw and cooked meat.
- Regularly checking that fridges are below 5 degrees centigrade and freezers are below minus 18 degrees centigrade.
- Paying attention to date codes on bought food.
- Ensuring fish, poultry and meat are completely defrosted before cooking, and are cooked right through.

- Not refreezing thawed food.

Appendix F: Example Of A Client Session

Client: 44 year old woman. Has asthma and dry skin. Feels she is taking a lot of supplements and isn't sure they are doing her any good. Wants to "eat more healthily" but not very good at sticking to things.

Q: Would it be appropriate to do some questioning around diet and supplements? Yes
Q: Would it be appropriate to use the nutritional testing menu? Yes
Q: Is the first thing we should look at on the first page? No
Q: Is it on the second page? No
Q: Is it on the third page? No
Q: Is it on the fourth page? Yes
Q: Is it fibre? No
Q: Is it protein? No
Q: Is it oils and fats? Yes
Q: Is it saturated fats? Yes
Q: Does Sue need to decrease her intake of saturated fats? Yes
Q: is it in general? Yes
Q: by how much – at least 50%? Yes
Q at least 60%? No
Q: so, between 50% and 60%? Yes
Q: Do we need to be more exact than that? No
Q: so, is there anything else we need to know about saturated fats for Sue? No
Q: Is there anything else we should look at from the menu? Yes
Q: Is it on the first page? No
Q: Is it on the second page? Yes
Q: Is it snacking? No
Q: Is it timing? No
Q: Is it Food Quality? No
Q: Is it Food Storage and Preparation? Yes
Q: Is it about temperature? Yes
Q: Is it about the settings for her fridge or freezer? No
Q: Is this all food? No
Q: Is it one particular food or category of foods? Yes
Q: so, is it a single food? No
Q: Is it a category of foods? Yes
Q: What is the best way to find this category? Is it a culinary category? No
Q: Is it a nutritional category? No
Q: Is it a food family? Yes
Q: is it on the first page of the food families list? Yes
Q: Is it fungi/moulds? No
Q: Grasses? No

Q: Lily family? No
Q: Mustard family? Yes.

I read out to Sue all the foods in that food family – she asked if I could write them down for her so I did. I asked her how she stored these. She told me that she kept watercress in the fridge, mustard and cress on the window ledge and cabbage in a box under the sink (she doesn't like any other members of this food family.)

Q: Should all the members of the family be stored in the same way? Yes
Q: Is it sufficient for her to keep them in the fridge? Yes
Q: Is there anything else we need to know about temperature at the moment? Yes
Q: Is it about the mustard family? No
Q: Is it about another food family? Yes

I then work out which family it is, etc.
Once this is done:

Q: Would it be appropriate to do more on the nutritional menu now? Yes

I question as before to find the correct topic. In this example supplements have come up.

Q: Is it supplements? Yes

Sue is taking Company X's Zinc; Company Y's Multivitamin and Minerals With Iron, and Company Y's evening primrose oil supplement.

Q: Is the zinc supplement beneficial? Yes
Q: Do we need to change anything about it? Yes
Q: Is it to do with the amount she takes? No
Q: Is it to do with when she takes it? – spongy response
Q: Is it about what she has at the same time? Yes
Q: So is there something she should avoid when she takes the zinc? Yes
Q: Is it drinking tea at the same time? Yes [See page 118 for why I ask this question. If you did not know or remember this information, you could still arrive at this answer by asking systematic questions.]
Q: so when she takes the zinc, how far away should the tea be? Is it the same before and after? Yes.
Q: Is it at least one hour? Yes
Q: Does it need to be more than that? No

I check for allergy, tolerance and vital energy and all are fine.

Q: Is there anything else we need to know about the zinc? No
Q: Is the multi-vitamin supplement beneficial? No
Q: Is it harmful? Yes
I told Sue she should stop this immediately as it is harmful to her.

Q: Is the EPO supplement beneficial? Yes

I check for allergy, tolerance and vital energy and all are fine.

Q: Is there anything else we need to know about the EPO supplement? No
Q: Is there anything else we need to know about supplements? Yes
Q: Does Sue need to add an additional supplement? Yes
Q: Is it one I have here? Yes
Q: Is it in the Lambert's test kit? Yes
Q: In the first box? Yes
Q: Is it in this row? No.
Q: This row? Yes

I asked about each one in the row and got 8029 Vitamin B-50 complex.

Q: Does Sue take it according to the bottle? Yes

I check for allergy, tolerance and vital energy and all are fine.

Q: Is there anything else we need to know about the Vitamin B complex? No
Q: Is there anything else we need to know before we stop? Yes
Q: Is it when we should review this again? Yes
Q: Is it at the next appointment? Yes
Q: Do we now have energy permission to stop? Yes

Jane Thurnell-Read is a former university lecturer in sociology and management studies. For over 20 years she worked as a complementary therapy practitioner. She also taught students and therapists in USA, Belgium, Germany, Switzerland and Russia, as well as the UK. She was on the board of directors for the UK Kinesiology Federation, the professional association for her practice.

She has published 5 other books and written numerous articles on health and therapies. She has also been interviewed for television and radio.

She has a very successful business selling testing kits online to therapists worldwide. She also publishes three other web sites: one specifically for therapists, one for the general public on health and happiness (including an online shop selling healthy living products) and one for beginners and enthusiasts on sport and fitness.

Printed in the United Kingdom by
Lightning Source UK Ltd., Milton Keynes
137081UK00001BB/59-428/P